Slimming World

*fast*food

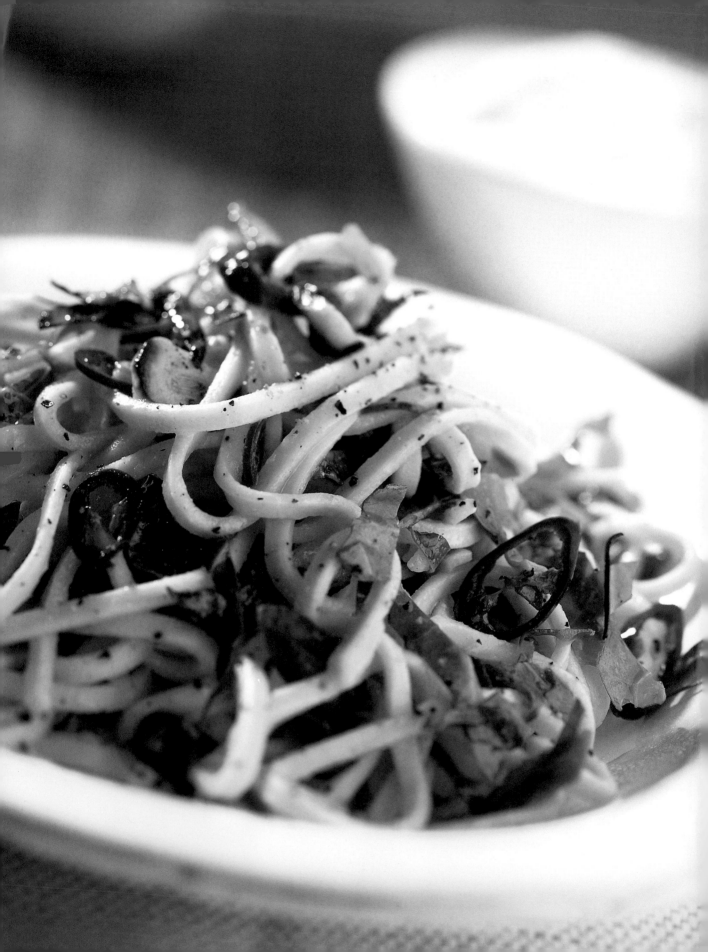

Slimming World

*fast*food

quick, delicious recipes to help you
lose weight and feel great

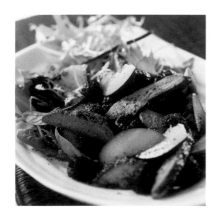
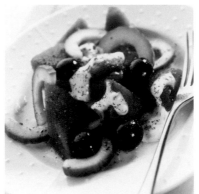
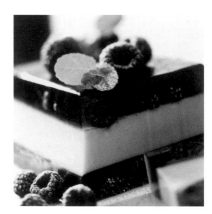

INDEX

This edition published 2003 for Index Books Ltd

First published in 2002

1 3 5 7 9 10 8 6 4 2

First published by Ebury Press
Random House, 20 Vauxhall Bridge Road, London SW1V 2SA

Random House Australia (Pty) Limited
20 Alfred Street, Milsons Point, Sydney, New South Wales 2061, Australia

Random House New Zealand Limited
18 Poland Road, Glenfield, Auckland 10, New Zealand

Random House South Africa (Pty) Limited
Endulini, 5a Jubilee Road, Parktown 2193, South Africa

The Random House Group Limited Reg. No. 954009

www.randomhouse.co.uk

A CIP catalogue record for this book is available from the British Library

Project editor: Janet Illsley
Recipes created by Sunil Vijayakar
Design: Anne-Marie Bulat and Liz Brown

Food photography: Ian O'Leary
Food stylist: Sunil Vijayakar
Prop Stylist: Helen Trent

FOR SLIMMING WORLD
Founder and Chairman: Margaret Miles-Bramwell
Managing Director: Caryl Richards
Project co-ordinator: Allison Brentnall
Text by Christine Michael

Printed and bound by Tien Wah Press Pte Ltd

Slimming World

Founded in 1969 by Margaret Miles-Bramwell, Slimming World is the UK's most advanced slimming organisation. It currently manages thousands of classes across the country with over 250,000 members attending every month, and another 15,000 attending free as successful target members. Each week, around 2,000 members reach their personal target weight. The astonishing success of Slimming World's Food Optimising is legendary.

cookery notes

- Both metric and imperial measures are given for the recipes. Follow either set of measures, not a mixture of both, as they are not interchangeable.

- All spoon measures are level: 1 tsp = 5 ml spoon, 1 tbsp = 15 ml spoon.

- Ovens should be preheated to the specified temperature. Grills should also be preheated. The cooking times given in the recipes assume that this has been done.

- Use large eggs except where otherwise specified. We recommend the use of organic or free-range eggs.

- Note that some of the dessert recipes contain raw or lightly cooked eggs. Avoid serving these to anyone who is pregnant or in a vulnerable health group, because of the small risk of salmonella infection.

- Always use fresh herbs, unless dried herbs are suggested in the recipe.

- Use freshly ground black pepper and sea salt unless otherwise specified.

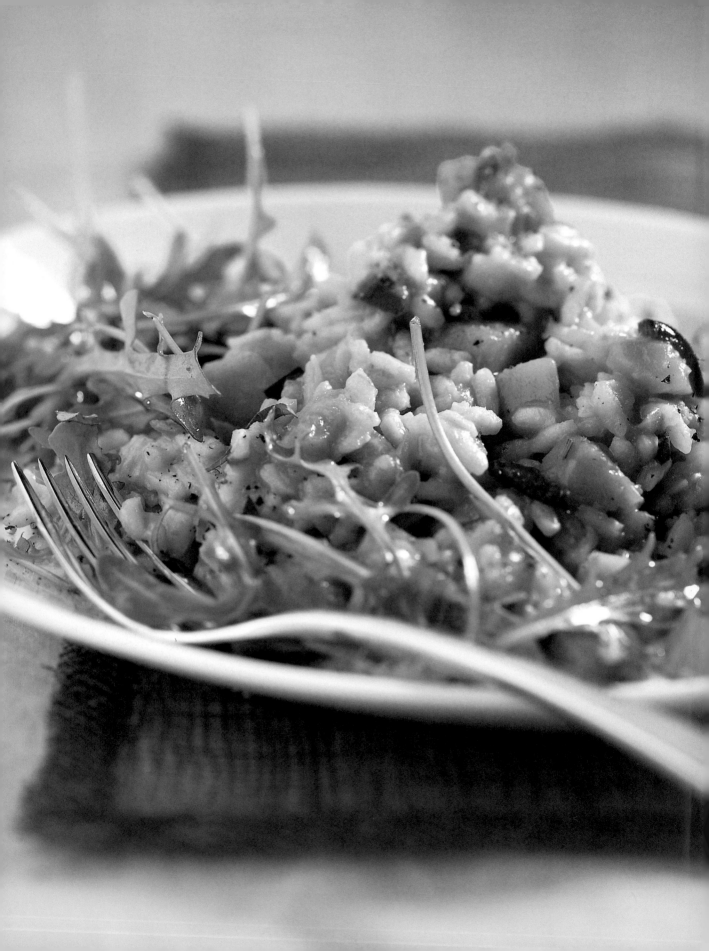

contents

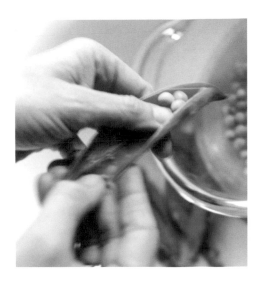
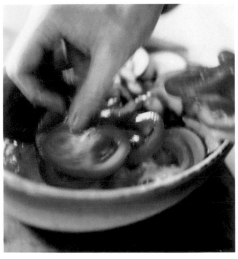
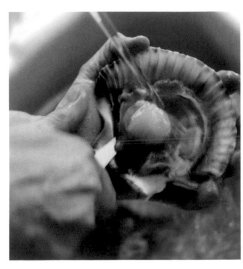

Foreword

Dear reader,

At Slimming World we always say there are no strangers; only friends you haven't yet met. You and I may not have met personally, but thank you for allowing us the chance to spend a few moments together as you open this book.

In many ways, although it may sound presumptuous, I feel as if I am talking to you as a friend, because friends have things in common. If you have ever longed for a slim body that doesn't put on an ounce, for example, I'm right there with you. If you have ever dreamed of finding a 'magic bullet' to solve your weight problem at a stroke, you're not alone. And if you feel that you want to be slim but don't want to make any changes to your lifestyle, I find that totally understandable, too.

And that is why I am delighted to share with you this wonderful system of Food Optimising which, as an everyday slimmer and a food lover, I know to be the most generous, most effective, and most flexible weight loss system possible. Hundreds of thousands of men and women have used Food Optimising, lost weight by it and continue to live by its principles.

With Food Optimising you will discover that, in order to be slim, there are changes to be made, but those changes needn't be as drastic as you might imagine. What's more, you can be confident that when you Food Optimise you are losing weight in the way that's known to be the healthiest and safest there is, in line with the latest nutritional thinking.

And Food Optimising is about far more than food! More than 30 years' experience at Slimming World has taught us that losing weight successfully is about motivation, enjoyment, and lightening the burden of unnecessary guilt and other negative feelings that we slimmers are prone to saddle ourselves with.

So thank you, once again, for deciding that you would like to explore Food Optimising with this book; we at Slimming World are honoured that you have made this commitment to us. And should you decide that changing your size is important to you, or that you'd love to overcome a troublesome weight problem and become the person you've always longed to be, then I hope you know that your friends at Slimming World will do all in our power to make those dreams come true.

Warmest wishes,

Margaret Miles-Bramwell
Founder of Slimming World

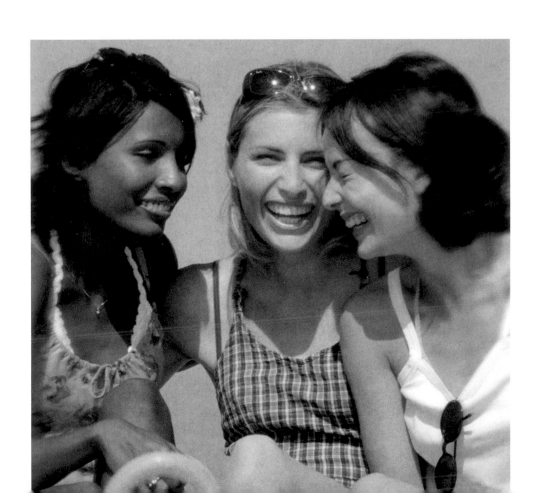

The Food Optimising concept

If you are one of the millions of people in this country who struggle with their weight, you may open this book with mixed feelings. Everywhere you look these days, you are bombarded with advertisements for the latest 'miracle diet', promising the solution you've been searching for. You may have tried different ways of losing weight and been disappointed, either because they didn't work for you, or because the effects lasted only a short time.

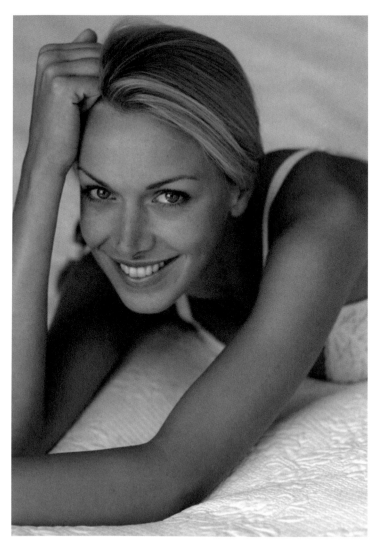

Certainly, you may wonder whether this collection of recipes, devised using Slimming World's Food Optimising system, could be any different. And the answer that you would hear, loud and clear if you attended one of the thousands of Slimming World classes held across the country each week, would be: 'Yes, yes, yes!'

What is it about Food Optimising that gets people so enthusiastic that they want to tell the world how it's changed their lives? On one level the answer is simple: it's a way of losing weight without ever needing to go hungry, and without feeling deprived of the foods you enjoy. But on a deeper level, Food Optimising is much more complex. It is based on 30 years' experience of how over-eating, dieting and healthy eating relate to each other in the real world, not in academic ivory towers or sterile laboratories. Although, of course, we respect and learn from everything that research and science can teach us.

Slimming World's philosophy is based on a deep understanding of how people with a weight problem feel, coupled with a passionate desire to help them achieve their goals. These principles were formed over 30 years ago and remain the bedrock of everything we do. Over the course of time, our unique and sophisticated Food Optimising system has been developed and refined in line with changing nutritional thinking. There is nothing faddy or 'weird' about Food Optimising. Follow the guidelines and you can be confident that the way you are eating is known to be healthy for people looking to lose weight today.

Being so close to slimmers for so long has enabled us to tailor Food Optimising exactly to your needs. Not only can you achieve your aim of losing weight, but you will also be eating to stay slim for life. Food Optimising offers you:

- A way of **eating to slim**, not starving to slim
- A way of **feeling free** and relaxed about food
- A way to slim while eating **normal**, **everyday meals** with your family
- A way of losing weight, while eating a wide range of **foods you enjoy**
- A way of satisfying your appetite so that you need **never go hungry**
- A way of knowing that you are **eating healthily** without having to worry
- A way of **enjoying your favourite treats** every day if you wish

Eating to slim, not starving to slim

The biggest difference you will notice when you start to Food Optimise, compared to other weight loss methods, is how much you can eat! Slimming World and Food Optimising are light years ahead of the 'cottage cheese and lettuce leaf' type of diet that was thought to be the only way in the seventies and eighties. When it comes to losing weight, many people still believe that 'if it's not hurting, it's not working'. Yet current thinking and Slimming World's own experience over the years, with hundreds of thousands of successful slimmers, is that the opposite is true.

Based on the scientific fact that to lose weight, you have to alter your 'energy balance' – in other words, you have to take in fewer calories than you expend – old-style diets were designed to cut calories drastically. Tiny portions of low-calorie foods were the order of the day, together with a strict ban on high-calorie favourites like cakes, chocolate and crisps. However, as many slimmers found, these diets were not only hard to follow, but counter-productive. The more you deprive yourself of comforting platefuls and favourite foods, the more you crave them, and the more likely you are to 'rebel'. Sooner or later, willpower crumbles, and you 'give in' to the foods you have been denying yourself with the result that the weight piles back on, and often some more besides.

Very low-calorie or 'crash' diets can also encourage an unhealthy relationship with food, and may have a damaging influence on your sense of worth and self-esteem. Since it is very difficult to stick to a crash diet for long, there will inevitably be times when you are 'on the diet' and times when you are 'off the diet'. This can lead to regarding certain foods as 'good' or 'bad', and to thinking about yourself as 'good' or 'bad', depending on what you are eating. The inability to stick to a restrictive regime comes to be seen as failure, for which you blame yourself, instead of blaming the diet for failing you!

Crash diets are bad for your physical well-being too. Cutting your food intake too drastically will result in losing lean tissue like muscle from the body, as well as fat. Since lean tissue processes energy efficiently, a loss of lean tissue can slow down your metabolism, making it even harder to process energy and lose weight. And as if that weren't enough, crash dieting can make it harder for your body to get all of the essential nutrients it needs.

For all these reasons, today's experts recommend gradual weight loss on a sensible calorie intake, rather than crash diets. And that's why Slimming World's Food Optimising turns all the old thinking about crash dieting on its head. We recognise that to lose weight healthily and comfortably, and to sustain that weight loss, slimmers need and want to eat lots of 'real' food, not diet food! They need to feel that they can fill their plates freely, to eat comfort food, and to enjoy their favourite foods, just like slim people do.

At Slimming World we understand the psychology of 'dieting' and we understand how important psychology is in providing a practical solution to the problems of overweight. The concept of **Free Foods** was formulated specifically to evade feelings of deprivation. We know it doesn't work to tell people that they can have as much salad (with fat-free dressing) as they want or that they should eat raw carrot when they're feeling peckish. Few slimmers enjoy salad or carrots to that extent and, in reality, vegetables on their own are not particularly satisfying.

Initially, to many diet experts, Slimming World's designated Free Foods seem quite outrageous – even some of our members are sceptical at first. Slimmers live most of their lives in fear of 'forbidden foods' and 'eating too much'. The notion that so many foods are now unrestricted is quite incredible. Won't slimmers just go overboard? Experience has shown us that they don't. If you can have Free Foods in quantity, you actually don't eat them in quantity. There is no need to deny yourself, or eat guiltily. You are freed from the fear of hunger, the urge to overeat disappears, and behaviour around food becomes much more rational. Decisions become real, not enforced; control comes from choice power, not cast-iron willpower.

So when we say fill your plate freely, we mean exactly that. With Food Optimising, you can eat as much as you like of a wide variety of **Free Foods**…as much as you like! This is the revelation that gets many people 'hooked'. Being able to **satisfy your appetite** on foods you love, and **still lose weight**, brings a feeling of freedom and a sense of joy to your weight loss journey that you previously thought impossible.

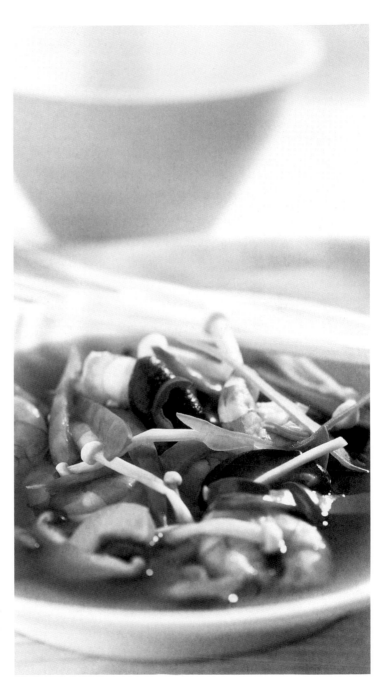

Lose weight, without counting calories?

By now, you will probably be wondering how Food Optimising can possibly help you take in fewer calories than you expend, which all the experts agree is the only way to lose weight. How can you control your calorie intake while you're piling your plate

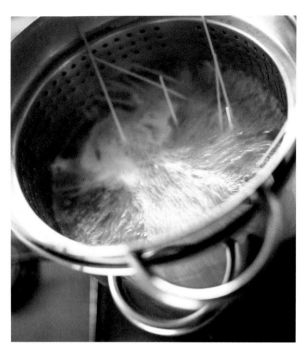

with pasta and potatoes? Surely you must have to count calories at some point? And how is it that Food Optimising allows you to eat unlimited amounts of foods that other diets almost always ban or restrict?

Put simply, Food Optimising is based on a scientific understanding of appetite, and how to satisfy it. It helps you to learn to make healthy food choices, which naturally limit your calorie intake – without counting a single calorie. It works like this: our appetite is controlled by many signals that arise as we chew, digest and absorb different foods. Some signals tell us to stop wanting more food when our body doesn't need any more (that's called **satiation**) and other signals prevent us from wanting to eat again until our body requires more energy (known as **satiety**). Scientific research has shown us that certain properties and components of foods make them much better at triggering these signals than other foods. Several years ago, Slimming World sponsored research into whether certain types of food had a greater satiation and satiety value than others. The results established that there was a hierarchy within the macronutrients – proteins, carbohydrates and fats. Proteins were found to lead the group, followed closely by carbohydrates and trailing well behind was fat. Foods rich in protein (for example, lean meat and fish) and those rich in carbohydrate (such as pasta and potatoes) are some of the most important in triggering these signals of satiation and satiety. Food Optimising shows you how you can eat your fill of these foods in order to satisfy your appetite and feel fuller for longer. This way, you naturally limit your overall energy intake and feel less need for high-sugar, high-fat snacks that pile on the calories (and the pounds) while providing little nutritional benefit.

Your lifestyle, your choice

Food Optimising recognises that while some people just love 'a meat-and-two-veg' roast dinner, or a full English breakfast, others prefer a big plateful of vegetable curry with rice, or a pile of pasta with tomato sauce. So Food Optimising is an eating plan that gives you a **choice** of two types of daily menu, **Green** and **Original** – designed to suit your tastes and lifestyle. Each day, you simply decide whether you want to have a Green or Original day, and stick to that choice all day. You can make every day a Green day, or have a mixture of Green and Original days. It's all about proportions. Some days you just fancy more meat and less potato, other days you look forward to lots of pasta or potato and much less meat. Any combination is catered for every day.

Whether you choose a Green or Original day, you will find there is a huge list of **Free Foods** for you to enjoy. Original day Free Foods include lean meat, bacon, poultry, fish and seafood, while Green day Free Foods include rice, pasta, beans and potatoes. Many foods, including eggs, fresh fruit and most vegetables, are Free Foods on both days, so you can make an enormous variety of delicious meals, whichever daily menu you choose.

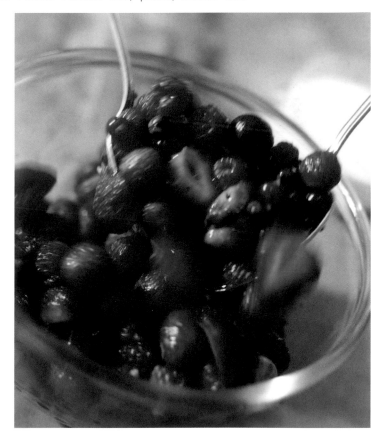

Then you get to eat some more! As well as all the Free Foods, every day we ask you to choose measured portions of **'Healthy Extras'** – more long lists of foods that boost your fibre, vitamins and minerals, especially calcium. These can include wholemeal bread, high-fibre breakfast cereals, soups and dairy products, and again you'll find there is a wide variety of foods to choose from. On Green days, the Healthy Extras list includes lean meat, fish and poultry, and on Original days, you could also choose potatoes, pasta or pulses.

And last but not least, there are those 'bits on the side' or treats, without which any diet would be hard to stick to. We know that only too well. And at Slimming World our light-hearted name for a little bit of what you fancy is 'Sins'. No food is banned at Slimming World, so it's up to you to choose how you use them and you'll find that high-Sin foods are typically those that are high in fat or sugar, or that don't have enough filling power for the amount of calories they provide.

But just as we don't tell you what to eat, we don't tell you how many Sins to have each day – it's your decision. Some days, with all the delicious Free Foods you've enjoyed, you'll be happy on as few as 5 Sins (for example, one glass of wine) and on others you'll need a more generous amount (such as a king-size Mars bar). For most people, an allocation of between 10 and 15 Sins a day is enough to keep the pounds rolling off, while still allowing a packet of crisps, or biscuits with morning coffee, every day they are 'on a diet'!

With other weight management systems, you have to know how many calories, grams of fat or some other kind of unit there is in everything you eat, before you eat it. With Food Optimising, you could easily fill up on delicious Free Food meals all day or all week without ever having to count a single Sin. Bliss!

You'll find more on the building blocks of Food Optimising later in this introduction. But as many thousands of people have discovered, who are happily eating more than ever before and losing weight more successfully than ever, you don't need to be a nutrition expert or worry about every detail for Food Optimising to work for you.

To see results, all you have to do is get started, and it really couldn't be simpler. Just choose your selection of **Free Foods, Healthy Extras** and **Sins**, and make up your own menus. With Food Optimising, we don't tell you what you must have for breakfast, lunch and dinner – as many weight loss diets do – you're in control all the way. To give you some ideas to get you started, we've suggested a selection of menus using recipes in this book.

Slimming World members quickly learn that they have plenty of choices. If you join us in class you'll soon be planning your own daily and weekly menus based on the foods you know that you will enjoy eating, and which will keep your appetite satisfied all day. You'll be amazed and thrilled at how good that feels, and how well it works … as you watch the pounds slip away.

One of the joys of this way of eating is that it is so flexible. People who associate 'dieting' with having to cook separate meals for themselves, and refusing invitations to eat out, find that Food Optimising is a glorious liberation from all that self-denial. It fits in with your lifestyle, whether you're out at work all day, catering for a family, entertaining friends or just cooking for yourself.

Do the family look forward to their Sunday roast every week? No problem: you can enjoy it with everyone else: just opt for a bigger portion of lean roast meat or dry-roast potatoes (depending on whether you've chosen Original or Green that day) and have loads of veg, topped with gravy (taken as Sins). Eating out with friends? Tuck into a smoked salmon and seafood starter, then a steak with jacket potato and vegetables, followed by strawberries (if you've got room). Fancy a snack when you get home from work? How about macaroni cheese, some fruit and a yogurt – before you even start to prepare supper!

Because Food Optimising is so flexible, it really is a way of managing your weight and eating healthily, which you can happily follow for life. Unlike a typical 'diet' which requires you to run your life around what you're allowed to eat, Food Optimising puts **you** in control. It is light years ahead of those diet sheets that you only stick to until you get bored with the menus, or decide that life is too short to give up your social life or all your favourite foods. As the principles of Food Optimising are based on the very best principles of nutrition, it's designed to work long-term to help you lose weight, and then to maintain a healthy, stable weight … forever. Welcome to the most advanced weight loss system ever. Welcome to Food Optimising.

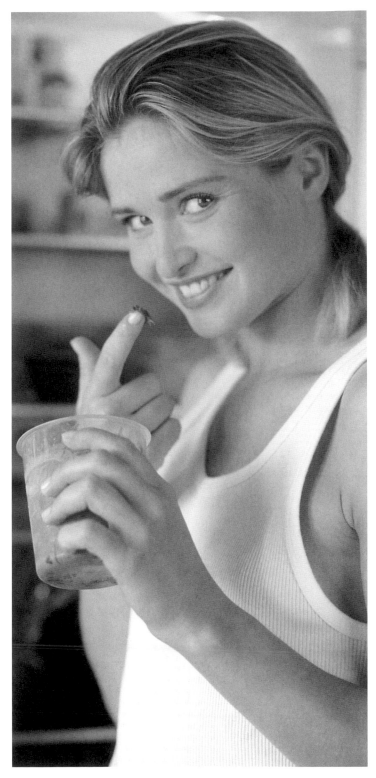

Food Optimising explained

Food Optimising doesn't entail strict rules, an in-depth knowledge of nutrition, or taking time to calculate what's in your food. The principles of Food Optimising take care of all that for you, so all you have to do is eat, enjoy, and lose weight. Once you have made Food Optimising a habit, you will find that it becomes second nature, fitting easily and comfortably into your lifestyle. But at this stage you may still have some unanswered questions, especially if you have been disappointed by weight loss methods you have tried before.

In this chapter, we present answers to questions often asked by newcomers to Slimming World. They will help you to understand the nutrition principles Food Optimising is based on, and how these work in practice to make it such an effective and enjoyable way to lose weight. If you join us at a Slimming World class, you will acquire lots more information and advice. You will also have the invaluable support and encouragement of your Consultant and fellow members, to inspire and motivate you to your chosen target weight – and help you to stay there for life.

Q *How can you 'pile your plate' with food, as you describe it, and still lose weight?*

A When you are Food Optimising, your plate will certainly be full – as full as you like – but the food that it is filled with will help you to lose pounds, rather than pile them on. A Food Optimising plateful will be **full of *less* energy-dense** foods (containing protein, complex carbohydrates and fibre) that keep you feeling fuller for longer; with only **small amounts of *highly* energy-dense** foods (fats, oils, sugar). Foods with a high energy density are those calorie-laden elements in your diet that have little nutritional benefit – often described as 'empty calorie foods'.

On a Green day, your plate will be full of unlimited potatoes, pasta or rice, with loads of vegetables and, if you like, a measured amount of lean meat or fish. On an Original day, your plate will also be piled high, with unlimited lean meat or fish, loads of vegetables once again, and a measured portion of pasta, pulses or potatoes.

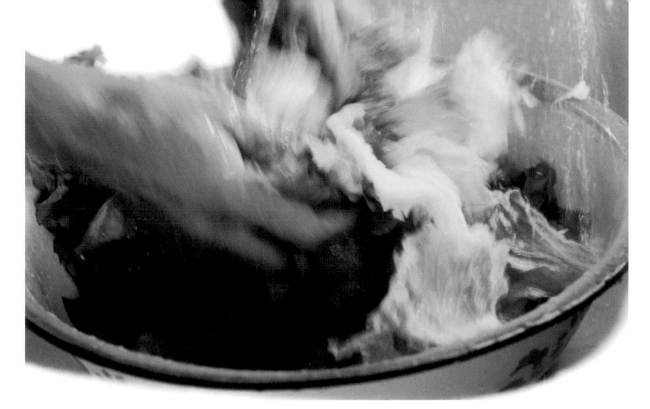

The abundant variety of foods that are **'free'** with Food Optimising are all foods that are **low in energy density** and **high in appetite satisfaction**. One of the most common remarks from successful Slimming World members is 'I can't believe how much I can eat and still lose weight!' And if you start Food Optimising, expect to hear: 'Are you sure you should be eating that much?' or 'I thought you were on a diet!'

Q *So what is energy density?*

A Energy density is the amount of calories contained within (or provided by) a specific weight of food. Energy density = calories per gram. So the weight of food we eat and how many calories that food supplies is described as the food's energy density. Foods that are high in energy density have a lot of calories packed into a small volume, they can be eaten quickly and lead to a high calorie intake within a short time. Foods that are low in energy density occupy a larger volume, take longer to eat, make you feel full and make it more difficult to consume a lot of calories. So, if you choose foods with low energy density you can still eat the same amount of food (or more) and feel satisfied, yet automatically reduce your calorie intake.

When you are Food Optimising, your body will recognise quickly the energy-giving, appetite-soothing carbohydrates and proteins and will send a clear signal to your brain: 'I can stop eating. I've had enough.' And because your meal is low in fat and sugar, your overall energy (calorie) intake will naturally be lower too.

Q *What difference does the amount of fat in a meal make?*

A Unlike carbohydrates and proteins, which are naturally filling or 'satiating', fat would seem to have the opposite effect. When we eat a high-fat meal or snack, our brain is likely to tell us 'More, more!' instead of 'I've had enough!' Our bodies just don't wake up to a large delivery of calories in the form of fat in the way that they do to a delivery of calories in the form of carbohydrate or protein – so we go on eating.

In terms of satiety, have a high-fat meal and you'll feel satisfied for a much shorter time too. When you're hungry again, you'll want a snack to keep you going. Choose a high-fat snack, like chocolate or crisps, and it's very tempting to keep on eating. Then because you don't feel full for long, the same thing happens, leading to a spiral of over-eating and weight gain. Many people in fact find that high-fat snacks, especially salty ones like crisps, are 'trigger foods'– they trigger a craving for more and more, without ever truly satisfying your hunger.

One of the problems with fat (and oil) is that it is highly energy dense. In other words, weight for weight (and usually volume for volume), fat has more than twice as many calories per gram as carbohydrate and protein. So when you eat a given amount of fat, you're taking in over twice as much energy (in the form of calories) than you would if you'd eaten protein or carbohydrate. Fat adds to the palatability of foods too, making them so much easier to eat! So no wonder it's easy to eat so much without your body realising how many calories it's taken in, a term described by scientists as 'passive over-consumption'. Add to this, the fact that even though you've taken in these excess calories, the high-fat foods don't keep you feeling satisfied after a meal, and you can see why protein-rich and carbohydrate-rich foods are far more useful from a slimmer's perspective.

This explains why people who start Food Optimising find that they seem to be eating much more than before, and yet losing weight. Swap a portion of meat pie and chips for a huge serving of lean meat with a jacket potato and vegetables and you will be eating more food, but the overall energy intake will be lower. So, too, will be your weight when you step on the scales at the end of the week. It seems almost miraculous that Food Optimising allows you to eat freely foods rich in protein or complex carbohydrates, yet it is scientifically proven that people consume far fewer calories overall when they eat this way.

Q *Sugar is a carbohydrate, so why isn't it free?*

A There are different forms of carbohydrates: starches (or complex carbohydrates) found in foods like pasta, pulses, rice and potatoes; and simple sugars such as those found in ordinary sugar, sweets and cakes. Both types, as we digest them, release sugars into the bloodstream. However, complex carbohydrates generally have a lower energy density than simple sugars. These foods usually contain plenty of fibre and water, which add bulk and volume to them without increasing the energy content, so lowering the energy density and helping us to feel full and satisfied without piling on calories.

Fibre also slows down the absorption and digestion of foods. In this way, the sugars are released into the bloodstream more gradually. The slow, gradual release of sugars into the bloodstream that we get from eating fibre-rich carbohydrates is thought to be more helpful in suppressing appetite than the 'sugar rush' we get from sugar itself and sugary foods.

Q *What about fruit and vegetables; don't they contain sugars too?*

A Yes, fruit and vegetables do contain carbohydrate in the form of sugars. But the sugars that occur naturally in these foods are a much better source of energy than the sugar in sweets and cakes, because they come with a whole host of important nutrients, including a variety of vitamins and minerals.

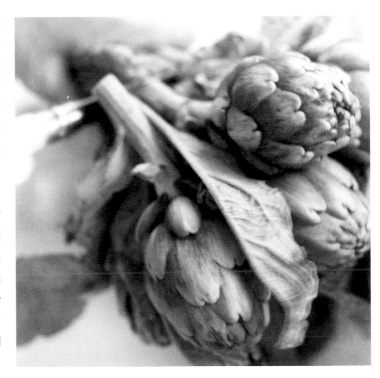

In fact, nutrition guidelines on healthy eating recommend that we eat at least five portions of fruit and vegetables each day. Fruit and vegetables also contain water and fibre, making them bulky, low energy-dense foods (effectively 'diluting' the calories) so they are great foods to fill you up while slimming.

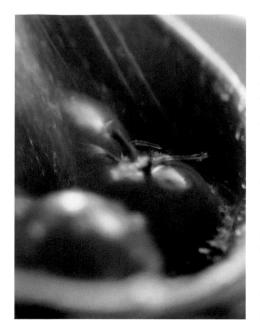

Processing foods can also have an effect on their satiating power. Whole fruits like apples, for instance, which contain fibre in the flesh and skin, have been shown to suppress your appetite more effectively than fruit juice or purée, from which the fibre is disrupted or removed. Compared with whole apples, apple juice and purée result in faster and easier ingestion and reduced satiety, making it easier to consume a lot more.

With Food Optimising, you are encouraged to eat whole fruit (low in energy density, and designated Free Foods) rather than juice or purée (higher in energy density, with Sin values), so you get maximum appetite satisfaction for minimum calories. Food Optimising encourages you to choose foods containing complex carbohydrates and fibre (less energy-dense foods), and to avoid quick fixes of sugary (highly energy-dense) foods, which may satisfy you initially, but will be followed by a rapid drop in your blood-sugar levels, leaving you wanting more.

Foods rich in complex carbohydrates include pasta, noodles and rice; potatoes; cereals and oats; bread; beans, peas and lentils; and grains, such as couscous and bulghar wheat. Most of these are **Free Foods** or **Healthy Extras** when Food Optimising, depending on whether you have chosen a Green or Original day.

Q *Where do proteins come in?*

A Protein-rich foods that are fairly low in fat include lean cuts of poultry, beef, pork, lamb and offal; fish; beans, peas and lentils; and other non-meat proteins such as Quorn and tofu. Depending on whether you have chosen a Green or Original day, most of these are **Free Foods** or **Healthy Extras**. As proteins are the most filling (satiating) of all the major food groups, having protein-rich foods in your meals will help you to eat less overall, as they fill you up and keep you satisfied for longer.

Q *Can I have meals that are high in both protein and carbohydrates?*

A Yes! Food Optimising is not about **separating** different types of **nutrients**, but about allowing you to choose the **proportions** of different types of **food you prefer**.

It allows you to fill up on the foods you elect to satisfy your taste buds and your appetite on that particular day, without having to worry about counting or measuring, and then adding other foods for balance. If you want to fill up on potatoes, pasta and rice (which contain lots of satiating complex carbohydrates), or perhaps beans, peas and lentils (which contain complex carbohydrates and are a good source of protein, too) then opt for the Green choice and you can do so freely. If on some days you feel like satisfying your appetite with lean meat, poultry or fish (rich in protein) then you can opt to choose an Original day. You can always add fruit and green vegetables (which contain some carbohydrate) to any meals quite freely on both Original and Green food days. By using Healthy Extras and Sins if you wish, you can have additional carbohydrate on an Original day, or protein on a Green day. And some non-meat proteins, like Quorn and tofu, are even Free Foods on Green days. In this way, your overall energy intake is reduced in an easy, stress-free and enjoyable way.

It's important to emphasise here that Food Optimising is not about 'food combining', where it is not permitted to eat protein-rich and carbohydrate-rich foods together in the same meal. With Food Optimising, depending on the type of day you choose, you simply have smaller portions of some foods, knowing that other really filling and great-tasting foods are on hand all day long. On a Green day, for example, you could choose a measured serving of lean mince in tomato sauce with loads of pasta (unlimited) to make a huge, tasty and very filling spaghetti bolognese. On an Original day, you could have a jacket potato, piled high with delicious, low fat chicken curry for a very satisfying lunch.

Q *How does Food Optimising give me enough fibre?*

A Food Optimising makes the most of fibre-rich foods, for the **least** amount of calories. For example, fruit and vegetables (low in energy density) are not only rich in fibre and a powerful protection against many diseases, they are also generally low in calories – and so they are **Free Foods** (unlimited) when you are Food Optimising. We suggest

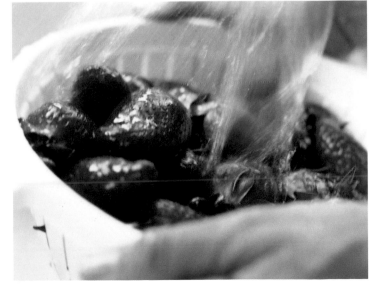

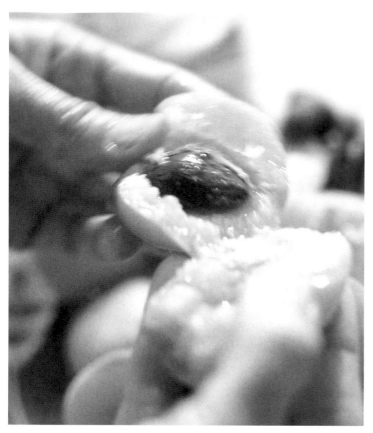

you eat at least five portions, or as many as you like, every single day. You will also discover that Food Optimising encourages you to choose high-fibre varieties of foods, such as wholemeal bread, wholemeal pasta and high-fibre breakfast cereals; and to add to the fibre content of meals such as casseroles, by including beans and lentils.

Having plenty of dietary fibre is a vital part of Food Optimising, not only because it is an excellent filler, but also because it is essential for good health. Eating plenty of fibre can protect against many illnesses, ranging from constipation to much more serious diseases, such as cancer of the colon and heart disease (by helping to reduce cholesterol).

When you start Food Optimising you may well find that you are eating more fibre-rich foods than you were before. If you know your current diet is low in fibre, we advise you to increase your fibre intake relatively slowly and to drink plenty of water; this is important for good health generally but especially for helping your body process fibre-rich foods.

Q What about Sins?

A 'Sin' is the light-hearted, humorous term we use to ridicule the idea that there is anything bad about food, or about anyone who enjoys eating all manner of foods. Foods on the Sin list are those that are too energy dense, or simply don't have the required filling power, to make losing weight easy. Sins are also the way that Food Optimising literally 'lightens the burden' for anyone who wants to shed the guilt, the self-blame and the self-punishment that so often accompany the 'dieting' process. Even today, some weight-loss organisations and some 'experts' give you the impression that breaking your diet, eating the wrong foods or eating too much is 'sinful' and that if you do not lose weight, you have only yourself to blame. Our approach to weight loss and weight maintenance is exactly the opposite. We want you to feel relaxed and light-hearted around food because you *need* to feel light-hearted and relaxed around food, for the sake of not only your sanity, but also your success – your ultimate, life-long, lasting success.

It's so important that we encourage you to have a 'Sin-a-day' as Slimming World's eating plan was first called. The ability to enjoy Sins with Food Optimising turns on its head the notion that some foods are 'good' or 'bad' (which incidentally is nutritionally wrong, as well as psychologically unhelpful). Including some Sins in your diet every day, while still losing weight successfully, is a great way to feel good about yourself, and keep your sense of humour. It is more effective than feeling 'good' because you've stuck rigidly to a diet that doesn't allow you any treats or fun.

As long as you're aware of how many Sins you're consuming – keeping a log of your daily Sin count is a good way to do this – and you stay within your chosen allocation, you will continue to lose weight. Remember that you choose how many Sins you'd like each day, so that you're in control. Some days it might be 5 Sins, others as many as 20 Sins. On a very special occasion such as a wedding, you might accept that it will be a 50- or even a 100-Sin day! Agree it with yourself in advance, keep counting and enjoy every one of those Sins on the day. The next day, get back to your normal chosen allowance, safe in the knowledge that you haven't 'blown it for good'. And there's no need to starve to make up for it, because you'll probably still lose weight. Although 50 or even 100 Sins sounds an awful lot in one day, it's undoubtedly fewer than if you'd stopped counting altogether, and certainly far less than if you felt you'd 'really blown it' and convinced yourself there was no point in even trying again.

Remember too that with Food Optimising, you only need count foods that you take as Sins. The vast majority of the food you will eat each day is **Free Food** – oodles of mouth-watering, satisfying and healthy foods that will fill you up and help you slim. Learning which foods can be eaten freely, and which foods need to be kept an eye on and counted, is a great way of learning how to eat healthily for life. And so liberating! An enlightening mix of control and free-wheeling that you can really enjoy. It's very different from calorie-counting, where you must count absolutely everything and stick rigidly within your daily limit. Focusing on foods that will be the kindest to your well-being, your happiness and your waistline is so much more positive.

Q *How much weight will I lose when I am Food Optimising?*

A Slimming World encourages a healthy rate of weight loss, averaging 500g–1kg (1–2lb) each week. This is a practical, achievable goal for the majority of people and encourages realistic expectations. Of course, everyone is different and people will lose weight at different rates – influenced by a number of factors such as genetics, how much weight someone has to lose, and how active they are. When people have quite a lot of weight to lose, it is not unusual to see quite large initial losses of 3–4.5kg (7–10lb) in the first week and more than 500g–1kg (1–2lb) in the following few weeks, which is partly due to the loss of water. We find, however, that with the majority of our members, weight loss settles to an average 500g–1kg (1–2lb) a week over time.

As part of Slimming World policy, we have discussed rates of weight loss with top medical advisors, who have confirmed that as long as people are Food Optimising properly, a rapid weight loss isn't a problem. As long as slimmers are eating plenty of food, having a balanced diet, and exercising to help maintain lean muscle tissue (which we would encourage), a weight loss of more than 500g–1kg (1–2lb) a week over several weeks, or even months, can still be perfectly healthy.

Losing weight too fast on too few calories is counter-productive, and you should never, ever crash diet. Crash dieting just isn't possible when you are Food Optimising – it's the most generous weight loss plan ever. Slimming World members regularly enjoy 1,500–1,800 calories a day. However, you may want to step up your weight loss at some point – perhaps it has slowed down and you don't know why. So Food Optimising includes Speed and Super Speed food choices. These Speed Foods contain even fewer calories (are even lower in energy density) compared to other foods of their type. Fill up on these and you will give your weight loss a boost.

Q *Will I have to exercise?*

A As with so many questions about weight loss and health, there is a short answer to this – and a much longer answer! The short answer is that it is perfectly possible to lose weight by changing your diet with Food Optimising, and without doing any extra exercise at all. If you go to a Slimming World class, you won't be asked to take part in a workout or aerobics session; we recognise that that isn't everyone's cup of tea. But there is a great deal of research to show that the healthiest way to lose

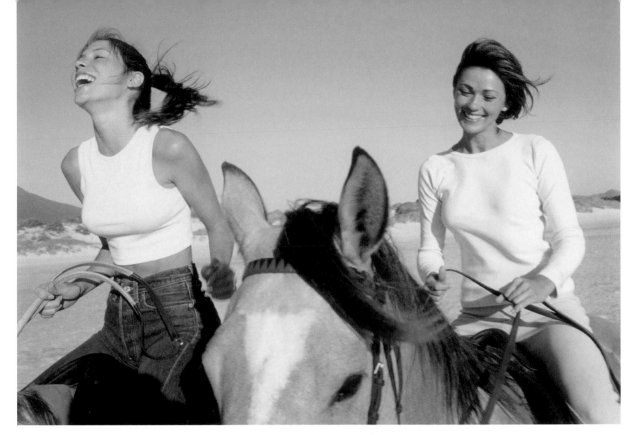

weight – and to keep it off in the long term – is to tackle both sides of the 'energy balance'. This implies a sensible reduction in energy intake (by Food Optimising) and a modest increase in energy expenditure (by becoming more active).

Taking some regular exercise doesn't necessitate joining a gym; it could mean a daily 15-minute walk around the block, taking the stairs instead of the lift every day at work, finding time for a swim a few times each week, or putting on your favourite music and dancing for 20 minutes every evening. The key is to find ways of becoming more active that don't involve radical changes to your lifestyle, so that they're easy to maintain and make a part of your daily routine.

Setting yourself small, progressive goals can be very helpful, such as a 5-minute walk every day for a week, then keeping this going or increasing it to 10 minutes for the next week, so that you can see what you are achieving. Choose an activity that you enjoy, and you may find that you want to start exercising more seriously, perhaps by going to a class or joining a group activity. But it's getting started that counts.

It's never too late to start becoming more active and the benefits of fitness are enormous, not only for your weight loss goals but also for your physical health and your general wellbeing. Becoming a regular exerciser, as well as a Food Optimiser, is another powerful tool to help you become slimmer, fitter, healthier and happier.

More than skin deep

Every culture and every era of history has had its own definitions of what it is to be physically beautiful. In the Western world, and at the beginning of the 21st century, the prevailing fashion is to be slim. This is by no means the custom in every part of the world, and in our own culture it was not fashionable as recently as a century ago. The 'slim is beautiful' world we live in is actually nothing more than a historical and cultural snapshot.

As other more enlightened cultures and periods of history have shown, being beautiful is about far more than your weight. But it can be hard to keep that sense of perspective and to hang on to your belief in your own personal beauty, when you seem to be swimming against the prevailing culture that says to be slim is to be beautiful and admired; to be overweight is to be ignored, discounted, disrespected.

When people are treated like this – for whatever reason – their sense of self-worth suffers a blow. Some weight management organisations and experts believe that the way to help overweight people become slimmer is to reinforce those negative feelings: to shame, blame and humiliate them into 'pulling themselves together'. Praise and support are partial: if you have a 'good week', you are rewarded; if you have a 'bad week', you are made to feel that you have not only failed personally, but have let others down as well.

Slimming World was formed as a result of a passionate belief that this is absolutely the worst way to motivate and encourage slimmers. Our philosophy is that people achieve most when their sense of inner beauty and self-worth is nurtured, not squashed. And in a culture where the odds are against them, overweight people do not need criticism and disapproval. On the contrary, they need consistent, constructive, caring support. At Slimming World, we call this support network 'IMAGE therapy'; it stands for Individual Motivation And Group Experience.

Unique to Slimming World classes, IMAGE therapy is based on 30 years' deep understanding of how it feels to be overweight and how hard it can be sometimes to feel that you are a person with unique and wonderful qualities, who deserves to be the very best you can be. For some people, learning about Food Optimising is the easy part; learning to rebuild their self-confidence and self-worth is harder, but ultimately just as rewarding.

What happens in class

Slimming World members attending their first class often remark upon how welcoming, warm and friendly it is. New members tend to go along with misconceptions, especially if they have had disappointing experiences with weight management organisations in the past. 'I thought it would be like school'; 'I thought everyone would stare at me'; 'I thought I'd be told off for having let myself get so big': these are just some of the worries that are quickly dispelled.

In fact, one of the surprises about joining Slimming World is that you can expect lots of praise and compliments before you've lost a single pound! That's because the people around you appreciate that just by stepping through the door, you have made a statement and a commitment that is worth applauding. And applaud you they will ... every time you lose weight; every time you share an idea you have that could help others; every time you have had a difficult week and come back to class anyway – knowing how much easier it is

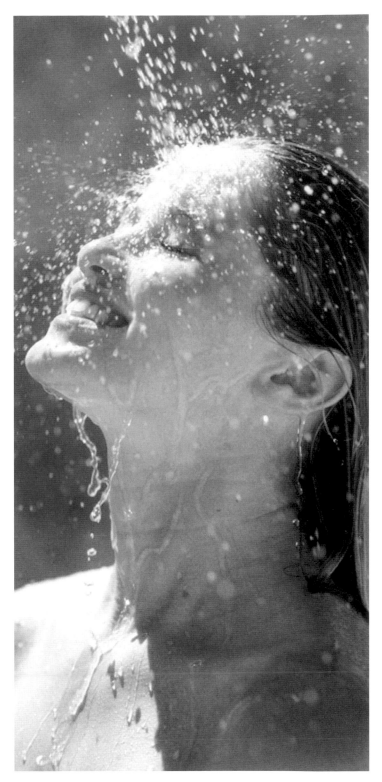

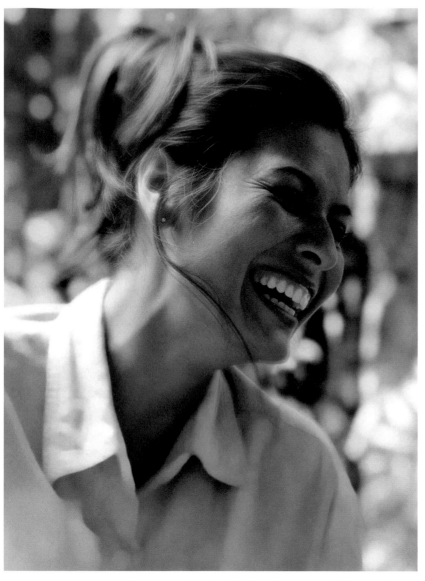

to stay away and come back next week. Deciding to come to class when you have slipped behind – to refuel your motivation and find the help you need – takes courage, and that's why it deserves praise.

Another surprise awaiting people who join Slimming World for the first time is that your Consultant is not a 'lecturer', telling you what to do and handing out rewards and punishments. Seats are arranged in a circle or horseshoe, and you'll soon realise that each individual member enjoys the support and warmth of the whole group – not just your Consultant or the people sitting nearest to you. It's wonderful to feel the power and the warmth of that support shining on you, showing you the way forward.

If your motivation is flagging, you will leave the class feeling valued, restored, and ready to start again. And if you went into class feeling positive and motivated, you will leave on an absolute high ... that's more delicious than any food!

If you're a shy, self-conscious person – like many people, in fact, who go to Slimming World – you might now be imagining that going to a class will be like joining some strange cult, and as a new recruit you'll be thrust into the spotlight! It isn't like that at all. For one thing, cults are not known for their sense of humour, whereas at a Slimming World class you'll probably laugh more than you would during a whole evening watching TV. And more importantly, you can participate just as much as you feel comfortable with; no one will single you out or embarrass you. (But don't be surprised if the liveliest person in the class takes you to one side to say that she refused even to take her coat off the first time she came!)

The aim of everything that happens in class is to increase members' awareness that they are worth far more than their weight, and to challenge the damaging perception that if you are overweight there is something wrong with you. Our mission in part is to help you see that you are able, imaginative, competent, funny, sexy, and more than equipped to control your life and your weight. Unlike the 'experts' who make you feel that you should be 'treated' or 'managed', Slimming World knows that you have it within yourself to make the changes you want to in your life. Food Optimising and IMAGE therapy are just two of the powerful tools that can help you do this, but the most empowering thought of all is that **you** are in control.

Losing weight is a process that can take some time, but changing the way you think takes no time at all. For example, think of yourself for a moment not as 'an overweight person' but as 'a slim person who is temporarily overweight'. How does that person feel, dress, behave, move, eat? Would thinking like that more often help you? At Slimming World we have over 30 years' experience of helping people to think more positively about themselves and empowering them to tackle the challenges in their lives more effectively.

YOU decide

We all know that we have to make decisions every day. Some are big, conscious decisions, like what colour to paint the bathroom walls. Others slip by almost unnoticed – but although they seem insignificant, they can change our lives. For example, when someone last criticised you, did you agree with them inwardly instead of challenging them? Or when someone paid you a compliment, did your mind instantly dismiss it as worthless instead of acknowledging it with pleasure? Why did you decide to react that way – and what effect did your decisions have on your self-esteem?

At Slimming World, we know how vital it is to be aware of the effects of the decisions we make – even the small, apparently insignificant ones that can have such devastating results. Many weight management systems take away your decision-making powers, by telling you what to eat and when to eat it. That's a bit like learning a foreign language in phrases on an audio tape; it's fine as long as you repeat what you've learned, but what happens when you're on holiday and you have to start making real conversations?

So when you join Slimming World we put **you** in charge of all the decisions – starting with the amount of weight you would like to lose. Your Personal Achievement Target, 'PAT' as we call it, is just that: it's up to you to decide the point at which you feel you would like to celebrate your success. Of course, if you feel, once you've got there, that you would like to set a new, lower PAT, that's fine too. But setting your own weight loss targets puts you totally in control of the process. It also takes away that awful negative feeling that you have 'failed' if you are just a few pounds short of a target that's been set for you, no matter how much weight you may have already lost.

'Starting small' can be much more effective than choosing a target weight that you haven't been since your teens. This is especially true if you have a lot of weight to lose. Medical evidence has shown that if you are very overweight, losing 10 per cent of your body weight can lead to significant health benefits, including an increase in your life expectancy. So a 10 per cent reduction in your weight is a milestone that we celebrate at Slimming World, with our 'Club 10' scheme.

Simply making a decision can be empowering in itself. Supposing, for instance, that you decided to join a Slimming World class that was taking place in a few days' time. For the rest of that week you might choose to eat more healthily in preparation – or you might decide to do exactly the opposite. Either way, the decision you had made to join the class would affect your behaviour, before you even went to the class itself.

If you join Slimming World you will learn a lot more about how you make decisions, and the consequences of what you decide. Each week you will be asked how much weight you would like to lose in the week to come, and if you will have any difficult choices to make, such as what to eat at a party. It's not about giving the 'right answers' and making the right decisions; it's more a question of being aware of the decisions that will help you achieve your weight loss goal directly, and those that will lead you to take the more 'scenic route'!

As you become aware of the decisions you are making every day, it becomes easier to take credit for the good ones, and responsibility for the less successful ones. For example, did someone really 'make you' eat that chocolate when you would rather have used your Sins on something else? Did you have that extra glass of wine because someone put you down and made you feel unhappy, or did you choose to accept their invitation to react in that way?

Living your life as a 'thermometer' – allowing other people to turn your emotional temperature up

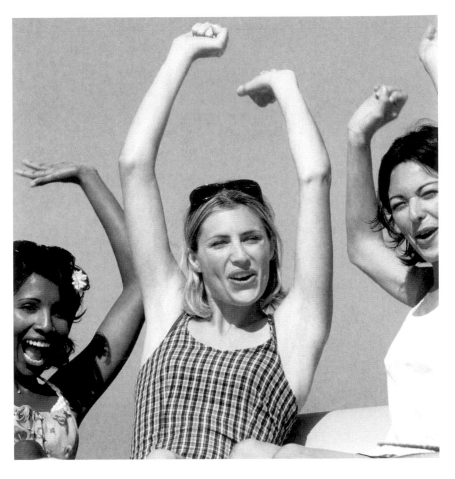

and down – is an uncomfortable way to live and makes it hard to manage your life, let alone your weight. Realising that you have the power to become a 'thermostat', by deciding how you will handle the variety of situations that confront you each and every day, is hugely liberating. For many people, it proves to be the key to managing their diet, and many other aspects of their lives, much more successfully than before.

Food Optimising is the powerful tool that frees you to experience the thrill of real control over your diet and your weight for life – IMAGE Therapy, and your Slimming World class, make it fun, and easier than you ever thought possible...

Food Optimising menus

Take a week or two to follow these varied, tasty menus, which feature some of the quick and easy recipes in this book. You will need to plan your shopping, and you'll be thrilled to find that Food Optimising works and that you can lose weight as easily as this.

The menus will help you understand the variety of meals that are possible with Food Optimising. They ensure you have enough good, nourishing food to keep you healthy and enable you to lose weight.

How to use Food Optimising menus most effectively:

• Decide whether you wish to have a Green or an Original day and stick to that choice all day. You can make every day a Green day, or include some Original days. Within the Green menus we've included meat-free choices suitable for vegetarians.
• Pick one breakfast, one lunch and one dinner from your chosen set.

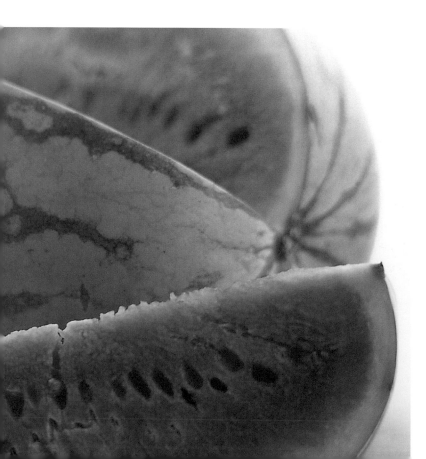

• Here's the fun bit – you can choose around 10 to 15 Sins' worth of food from the Sins lists (see pages 216–21). Some Food Optimisers find they lose weight most effectively on 5 Sins, others on 20 Sins. On some days, you might find you need to use 30. In general, we find 10 Sins a day is a good rule of thumb for effective weight loss.
• Check the foods on the menus that are highlighted in bold. These can be eaten **freely** without any weighing or measuring at all. Fill up on these foods whenever you feel peckish. You can also turn to our Free Foods list (see page 220) and select other Free Foods to enjoy whenever you want, in whatever quantity you want.

To maximise your healthy eating:

- Eat at least five portions of fresh fruit and vegetables every day. Frozen and canned vegetables can also be used.
- Trim any visible fat off meat and remove any skin from poultry.
- Vary your choices as much as possible to ensure the widest range of nutrients in your diet.
- Eat at least 2 portions of fish a week, of which one should be oily fish (unless, of course, you are a vegetarian).
- Try to avoid eating more than 10 eggs per week as these are particularly high in cholesterol. People with high blood cholesterol are advised not to eat more than 4 eggs per week although each individual should check with their doctor.
- Aim to keep your salt intake to no more than 6g a day (about 1 level teaspoon). As well as limiting the amount of table salt you add to food, watch out for salt added to manufactured foods and sauces. Try flavouring foods with herbs and spices instead.
- Remember the latest recommendations regarding intake of fluids which is to aim for 6–8 cups, mugs or glasses of any type of fluid (excluding alcohol) per day.
- Choose a milk allowance each day from the following:

   350ml/12fl oz skimmed milk

   250ml/8fl oz semi-skimmed milk

   175ml/6fl oz whole milk

   250ml/8fl oz calcium-enriched soya milk, sweetened or unsweetened
- *Or* if you prefer cheese rather than milk, choose a cheese allowance from the following:

   30g/1oz Cheddar

   30g/1oz Edam or Gouda

   40g/1½oz Mozzarella

   40g/1½oz reduced fat Cheddar or Cheshire

   3 triangles Original Dairylea (not chunky)
- Drink black tea, coffee (sweetened with artificial sweetener) and low-calorie drinks freely, and use fat-free French or vinaigrette-style salad dressings freely.
- Note that Healthy Extras are built into the menus.

When you have experienced the pleasure of Food Optimising on your plate, you will want to make your own menus. You can do this with the complete Food Optimising system, which is available at Slimming World classes throughout the UK.

Green menus

BREAKFASTS

- Fresh **melon** wedges
  followed by
  30g/1oz Honey Nut Shredded Wheat
  served with milk from the allowance and
  topped with fresh **strawberries**

- Two small slices wholemeal bread,
  toasted and topped with **spaghetti
  hoops** or **baked beans** in tomato sauce
  followed by
  an **apple** and a **banana**

- Omelette filled with grilled **mushrooms**,
  tomatoes and 40g/1½oz reduced fat
  Cheddar cheese, grated, and served with
  baked beans
  followed by a **banana**

- Fresh **grapefruit** sweetened with artificial
  sweetener if desired
  followed by
  40g/1½oz Nestlé Fibre 1 with milk from
  the allowance and a pot of **Ski Light
  virtually fat-free yogurt**

- 300g/10oz apple and 300g/10oz rhubarb,
  stewed with artificial sweetener, cooled
  then layered with **very low fat natural
  fromage frais**, sweetened with artificial
  sweetener and sprinkled with nutmeg

- Kedgeree: sliced **onion** fried with a pinch
  of curry powder using a little Fry Light,
  then mixed with boiled **rice**, 150g/5oz
  flaked poached haddock and a
  quartered hard-boiled **egg**
  followed by an **apple**

- 30g/1oz bran flakes topped with
  raspberries and served with milk from
  the allowance
  followed by a **pear** and a **satsuma**

- Soft-boiled **eggs** with 'soldiers' cut from
  2 small slices wholemeal bread
  followed by
  a fresh **fruit salad** topped with a
  Müllerlight yogurt

- Yogurt crunch made with **very low fat
  natural yogurt**, 30g/1oz Jordan's Luxury
  Muesli and sliced **kiwi fruit**: layer the
  kiwi, muesli and yogurt in a tall glass,
  finishing with a slice of kiwi
  followed by
  1 Allinson wholemeal crispbread topped
  with sliced **banana**

- 85g (3 rashers) grilled lean bacon, a
  poached **egg**, grilled **tomatoes** and
  mushrooms
  followed by a **peach**

LUNCHES

- French-style ratatouille (see page 161)
  followed by
  300g/10oz blackberries, stewed without sugar and topped with **very low fat natural yogurt**

- **Jacket potato** filled with 40g/1½oz grated reduced fat Cheddar cheese and **baked beans** in tomato sauce, served with lots of **salad**
  followed by
  an **apple** or **banana**

- Orange and ginger noodles (see page 148)
  followed by
  350g/12oz pears canned in natural juice, topped with **very low fat natural fromage frais** sweetened with artificial sweetener

- **Creamy dal** (see page 169), served with boiled **rice**
  followed by
  400g/14oz fruit cocktail canned in natural juice

- 85g/3oz smoked salmon, served with **Baked stuffed herbed tomatoes** (see page 165) and new **potatoes** cooked with fresh **mint**, plus lots of **salad**

- **Jacket potato** filled with 115g/4oz tuna canned in brine, and **sweetcorn**, served with a salad of **radicchio**, **endive**, **radishes** and cherry **tomatoes**
  followed by
  Müllerlight toffee yogurt sprinkled with ground cinnamon

- Fennel and wild rice salad (see page 174)
  followed by
  strawberries and **raspberries** layered with **Müllerlight vanilla yogurt** and sprinkled with 20g/¾oz chopped mixed nuts

- 60g/2oz wholemeal crusty roll filled with scrambled **egg** and sliced **tomato**
  followed by
  fresh **strawberries** topped with **very low fat natural yogurt**

- Pasta salad made with **pasta** shapes, cherry **tomatoes**, chopped **peppers**, **cucumber**, **sweetcorn** and freshly chopped **basil**, mixed with **Quark** flavoured with freshly chopped **garlic**
  followed by
  350g/12oz apricots canned in natural juice, topped with **very low fat natural fromage frais** sweetened with artificial sweetener

- 115g/4oz skinless, boneless chicken breast, grilled until tender and served with **Spiced roasted baby new potatoes** (see page 170) and **baby corn, mangetout** and **broccoli**
  followed by
  a **pear** and a **banana**

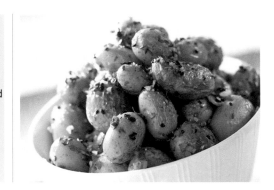

DINNERS

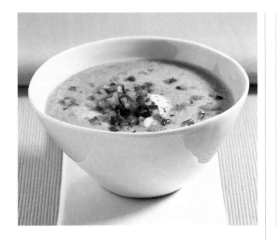

- **Creamy gazpacho** (see page 67)
  followed by
  Jewelled tabbouleh (see page 152)
  followed by
  a bowl of fresh tropical fruit salad: chopped **mango, kiwi fruit** and **papaya**

- **Penne arrabiata** (see page 141), served with a large mixed **salad**
  followed by
  an **apple** and a **satsuma**

- Vegetable stir-fry: **broccoli** and **cauliflower** florets, chopped **carrots**, mixed **peppers**, spring **onions**, button **mushrooms, beansprouts** and **waterchestnuts**, stir-fried with **garlic, herbs** and **soy sauce**, and served on a bed of **bulghar wheat** or **couscous**
  followed by
  an **apple**

- **Omelette** filled with chopped **peppers**, red **onions** and **sweetcorn**, served with **Herb and sweet potato rosti** (see page 132) and lots of **salad**
  followed by
  half a canteloupe **melon** filled with **raspberries**

- **Special vegetable fried rice** (see page 157)
  followed by
  very low fat natural fromage frais flavoured with vanilla and mixed with sliced **banana**

● **Jacket potato** filled with mixed **beans**, served with lots of mixed **salad**

followed by

strawberries and **very low fat natural fromage frais** sweetened with artificial sweetener and flavoured with vanilla

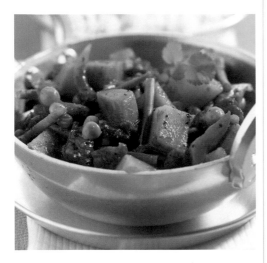

● Vegetable balti (see page 138) served with boiled **rice**

followed by

a bowl of chopped **apple, pear** and **grapes** topped with **very low fat natural yogurt**

● **Bean and mushroom burgers** (see page 136) served with a jacket **potato** and lots of **salad**

followed by

an **apple** and an **orange**

● **Vegetable chow mein** (see page 149)

followed by

mixed fresh **berries** topped with **very low fat natural fromage frais** sweetened with artificial sweetener and flavoured with vanilla

● **Aubergine pâté with crudités** (see page 48)

followed by

Grilled vegetables with herb salsa (see page 54) served with **Quorn chunks**

followed by

a **banana**

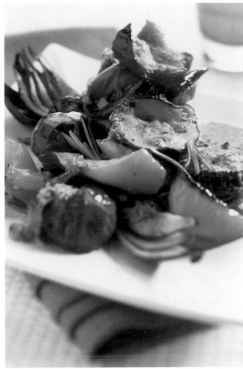

Original menus

BREAKFASTS

- Fresh **grapefruit**
  followed by
  lean grilled **gammon**, poached **egg**,
  grilled **tomatoes** and **mushrooms** served
  with 2 small slices of wholemeal toast

- 40g/1½oz Kellogg's All Bran, served with
  milk from the allowance, and topped
  with sliced **banana**, plus a pot of
  St Ivel Shape custard-style bio
  twinpot yogurt

- Chopped fresh **apricots**, with **very low**
  fat natural fromage frais sweetened with
  artificial sweetener, or **yogurt**
  followed by
  grilled lean **bacon**, scrambled **egg** and
  140g/5oz baked beans in tomato sauce

- **Bowyers 95% fat-free sausages**,
  served with grilled **mushrooms**,
  tomatoes, poached **egg** and 2 small
  slices of wholemeal toast

- 250g/9oz raspberries stewed with
  artificial sweetener, topped with a
  Müllerlight country berries yogurt
  followed by
  grilled **kippers**

- Banana split: **banana** sliced
  lengthways, sprinkled with 40g/1½oz
  Nestlé Fibre 1, and topped with **very low**
  fat natural yogurt

- 350g/12oz apricots canned in natural
  juice
  followed by
  an **omelette** filled with lean **ham** and
  mushrooms

- a slice of **melon**
  followed by
  boiled **eggs**, served with 2 small slices of
  wholemeal toast cut into 'soldiers'

- 30g/1oz Shredded Wheat Bitesize,
  served with milk from the allowance
  followed by
  grilled **kippers**, plus 1 Ryvita
  Original/Dark Rye/Sesame spread with
  Marmite

- Fresh **fruit salad**, such as **apple**, **pear**,
  green **grapes** and **orange**
  followed by
  grilled lean **bacon**, grilled
  tomatoes and **mushrooms**,
  served with 2 small slices of
  wholemeal toast

LUNCHES

- **Salmon** fillet baked with **coriander** and **lemon juice**, served with a large mixed **salad** and a 225g/8oz baked potato (raw weight)
  followed by
  a bunch of **grapes**

- **Mixed mushrooms with garlic, lemon and parsley** (see page 164), served with 100g/3½oz cooked wholemeal pasta
  followed by
  a **banana** and a **pear**

- **Grilled chicken and red onion salad** (see page 185), served with 200g/7oz new potatoes boiled in their skins, and a mixed **salad**
  followed by
  a **Müllerlight yogurt** and an **apple**

- Tuna salad: cherry **tomatoes**, diced **cucumber**, sliced **spring onion**, **cooked green beans**, chopped hard-boiled **egg**, and **tuna** canned in brine, mixed together and tossed with a little lemon juice and chopped parsley; served with a 60g/2oz wholemeal roll
  followed by
  fresh **strawberries** and cubes of **melon**

- Roast **turkey** breast served with **Cajun-style vegetables** (see page 168), and 200g/7oz new potatoes boiled in their skins
  followed by
  a **pear**

- **Duck, raspberry and peach salad** (see page 183) *followed by* 300g/10oz apple and 300g/10oz rhubarb stewed without sugar, topped with **very low fat natural fromage frais** sweetened with artificial sweetener

- 225g/8oz jacket potato (raw weight), filled with **very low fat natural cottage cheese** and chopped **spring onions**, served with lots of **salad**
  followed by
  apple and **orange** segments, topped with **very low fat natural fromage frais** sweetened with artificial sweetener

- **Herby mushroom and cheese turkey rolls** (see page 112), served with **baby corn, broccoli, carrots** and **mangetout**
  followed by
  400g/14oz fruit cocktail canned in natural juice

- **Grilled gammon steaks and tomatoes with herb mash** (see page 114)

  followed by

  225g/8oz apple, baked and served with 115g/4oz blackberries stewed without sugar

- **Prawn and chive omelette** (see page 81) served with 225g/8oz jacket potato (raw weight) and a large mixed **salad**

  followed by

  a **banana** and a **pear**

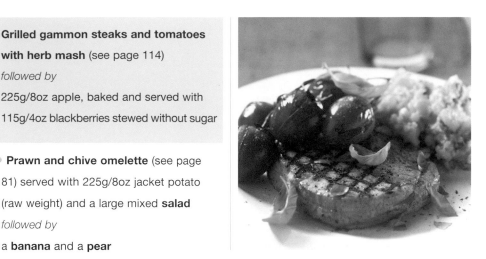

DINNERS

- Lean fillet **steak** tossed in crushed black **peppercorns**, grilled and served with **baby corn**, **sugar snap peas** and **asparagus**

  followed by

  fresh fruit salad, such as chopped **apple**, **banana** and **peach**

- **Seared tuna with hot pepper sauce** (see page 90), served with lots of **salad**

  followed by

  fresh **melon**

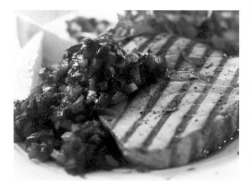

- **Spicy lamb steak** (see page 128), served with steamed **green beans**

  followed by

  raspberries and **strawberries**, topped with **very low fat natural fromage frais** sweetened with artificial sweetener

- **Italian chicken and tomato soup** (see page 73)

  followed by

  grilled lean **pork** steak, served with **swede**, **cabbage** and **carrots**

  followed by a **pear**

- **Prawns** sprinkled with **paprika**, served on a bed of crisp **lettuce** and **cucumber**

  followed by

  a grilled or baked **chicken** breast, served with **red cabbage**, thin **green beans** and **butternut squash**

- **Chargrilled Caribbean chicken** (see page 108), served with a green **salad**
followed by
a bowl of **raspberries**, **blackberries** and **blueberries**, topped with **very low fat natural fromage frais** sweetened with artificial sweetener

- **Honeydew melon**
followed by
Chive and ginger pork stir-fry (see page 118)
followed by
sliced fresh **mango** and seedless **grapes**, topped with **very low fat natural yogurt**

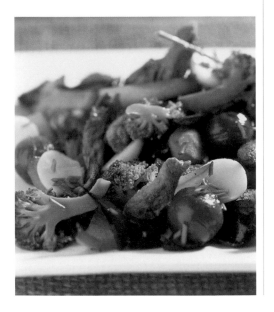

- **Tandoori monkfish** (see page 97), served with heaps of crisp green **salad**
followed by
a bowl of chopped **kiwi fruit** and fresh **pineapple**

- **Parma ham with minted melon wedges** (see page 64)
followed by
grilled **cod** served with **sugar snap peas**, **baby corn** and **carrots**
followed by
a **peach**

- **Grilled seafood skewers** (see page 60)
followed by
grilled lean **gammon** steak, topped with fresh **pineapple** chunks served with mixed **salad** leaves, cherry **tomatoes**, **cucumber**, **spring onions** and grated **carrot**

The Food Optimising storecupboard

When you are Food Optimising, you need ingredients at your fingertips that will enable you to produce a variety of quick, delicious meals, and help you lose weight. A good selection of spices and flavourings, for example, is essential to create a rich palette of flavours. Use the following list as a guide to useful standbys, and shop for fresh vegetables, herbs, fish and meat as you plan your meals.

- Canned products: tuna in brine or water; crabmeat in brine or water; sweetcorn niblets; borlotti, cannellini, red kidney and butter beans; chopped tomatoes (including the variety flavoured with garlic and herbs); black olives; water chestnuts; pineapple rings and peaches in natural juice; low fat coconut milk.
- Cooking mediums: spray cans of Fry Light (sunflower or olive oil based); olive oil and sesame oil (sometimes needed in tiny amounts to flavour a recipe).
- Spices and flavourings: sea salt, black and mixed peppercorns; coriander, cumin, caraway and fennel seeds; allspice and juniper berries; nutmeg, star anise, cloves, cardamom, cinnamon sticks; ground cumin, coriander, cinnamon, paprika, ginger, mixed spice, chilli powder; tandoori spice mix; curry powder; Cajun spice seasoning, dried chilli flakes; dried herbs, such as oregano; vanilla pods; saffron strands.
- Jars and bottles: Tabasco; Worcestershire sauce; sweet chilli sauce; passata; hoisin sauce; light and dark soya sauces; reduced sugar apricot jam; Thai fish sauce; reduced calorie mayonnaise; Dijon and wholegrain mustards; honey; capers and caperberries; gherkins; grated or creamed horseradish; mint jelly; chicken and beef Bovril; vegetable stock powder; balsamic, red and white wine vinegars; tarragon and cider vinegars.
- Staples: plain and wholemeal flours; long-grain, arborio, brown and wild rice; wholemeal and regular pasta, such as penne, spaghetti, linguini, parpardelle and fusilli; noodles; couscous and bulghar wheat; red lentils.
- Additional items: cornflour and arrowroot (to thicken sauces); artificial granulated sweetener; instant coffee granules; good quality chocolate; gelatine or vegi-gel, and sugar-free jelly crystals; meringue nests.
- Alcohol for cooking: red wine, dark rum, amaretto liqueur and marsala.
- Fridge items: very low fat fromage frais, yogurt and crème fraîche; Quark soft cheese; reduced fat cheese; Parmesan; eggs; skimmed or semi-skimmed milk; Quorn.

recipes

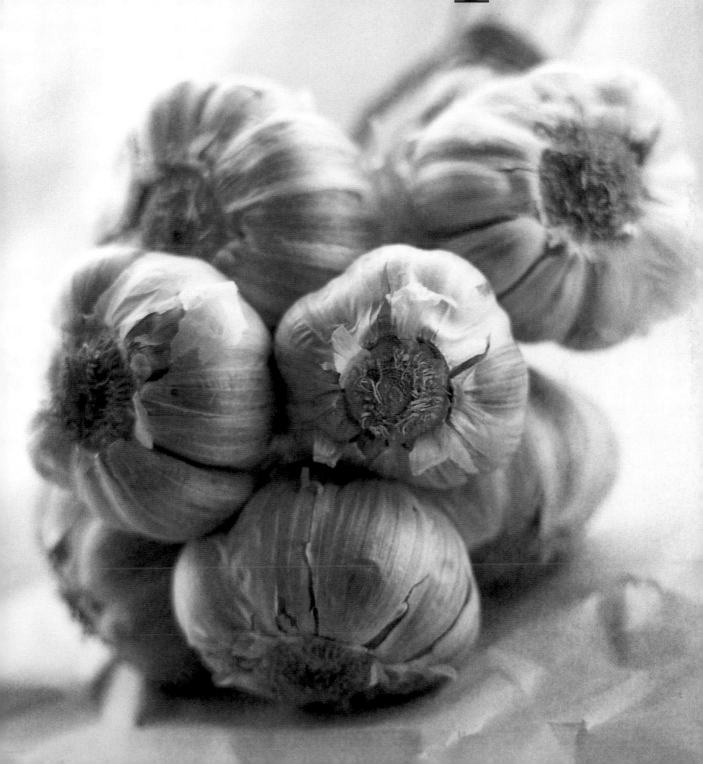

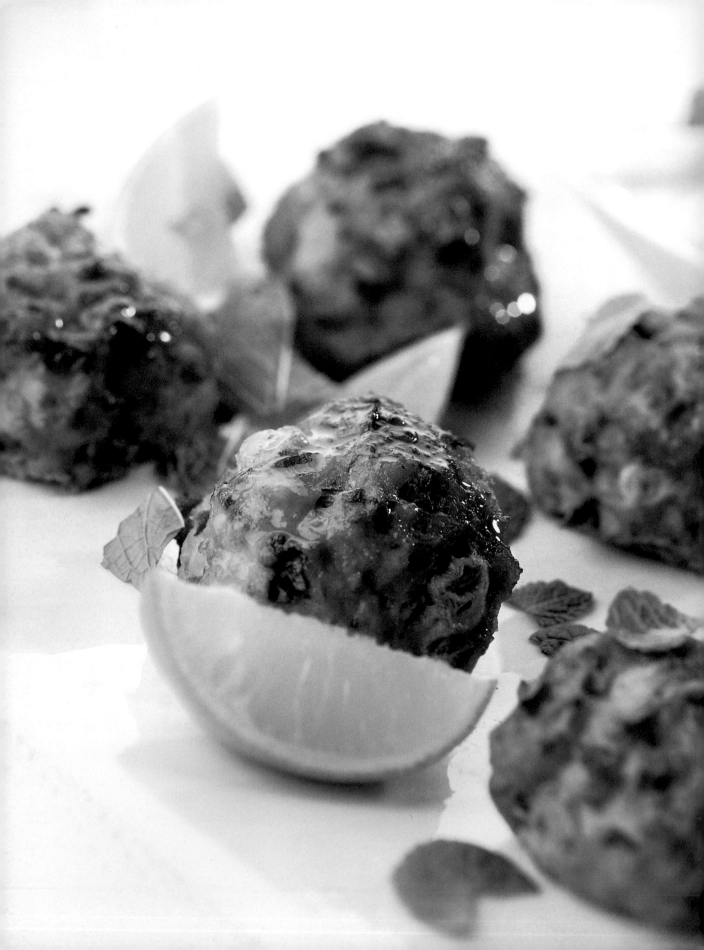

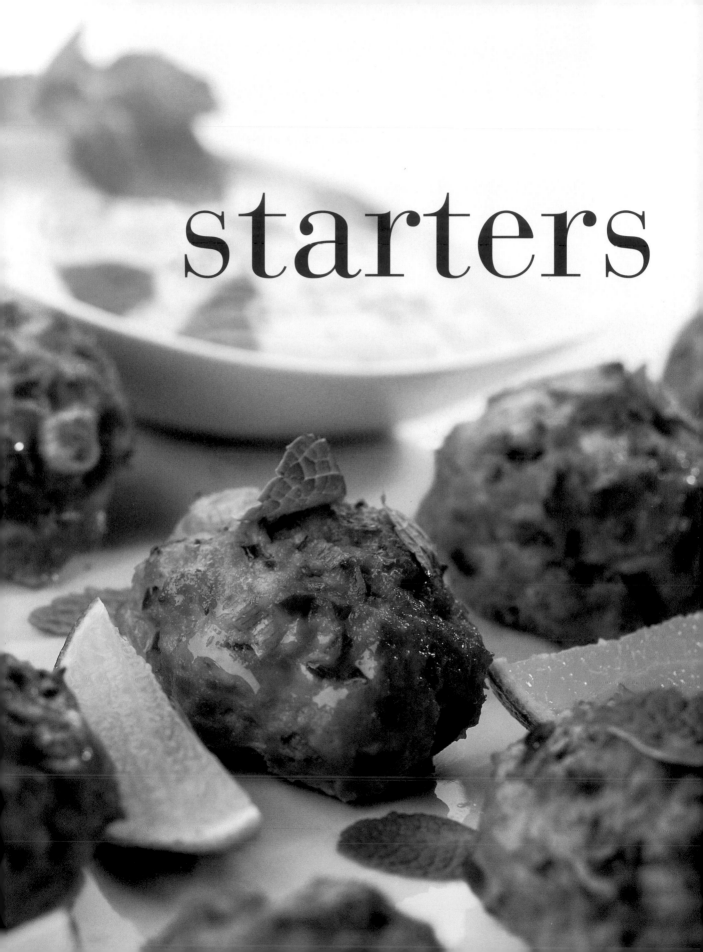

starters

Aubergine pâté with crudités

This creamy, herby pâté makes a great starter or healthy snack, and it's free on both Green and Original days. Just dip in and enjoy.

serves **4**

preparation

10 minutes,

plus chilling

cooking time

about 10 minutes

✓ vegetarian

2 large aubergines

3 garlic cloves, peeled and crushed

6 tbsp finely chopped mixed herbs (parsley,
    chives and thyme)

300g/10oz very low fat natural fromage frais

salt and freshly ground black pepper

FOR THE CRUDITÉS:

selection of crisp, raw vegetables chosen
    from the following:

red, green and yellow pepper slices

carrot sticks

celery sticks

cauliflower florets

radishes, trimmed

button mushrooms, trimmed

1 Cut the aubergines into bite-sized chunks. Add to a large pan of boiling water, bring back to the boil and cook for 10 minutes. Drain well and pat dry with kitchen paper.

2 Place the aubergine pieces in a food processor with the garlic and chopped herbs. Blend until smooth.

3 Transfer the aubergine mixture to a large bowl and stir in the fromage frais. Season well, cover and chill until ready to serve.

4 To serve, spoon the aubergine pâté into one large bowl or 4 individual ones and arrange your selection of vegetables around it.

Cook's note
You can use very low fat natural yogurt in place of the fromage frais.

original

Sin-free

green

Sin-free

Tomato, garlic and basil bruschetta

Bruschetta is the ultimate, quick and easy to prepare starter or snack. Our low fat version may not be Sin-free, but it's ideal for those who cannot resist this Italian treat. Try to use ripe, organic Italian plum tomatoes for maximum flavour.

4 large, thick slices crusty bread, each
   about 60g/2oz
2 garlic cloves, halved
3 ripe plum tomatoes

juice of ½ lemon
4 tbsp basil leaves, finely chopped
salt and freshly ground black pepper
basil leaves to garnish

1 Preheat the grill and toast the slices of bread on both sides until lightly browned. Rub one side of each slice with a cut garlic clove to impregnate the bread with the flavour and aroma of the garlic.

2 Dip the tomatoes into boiling water for 30 seconds, then remove and peel when cool enough to handle. Cut in half, scoop out the seeds, then roughly chop the tomatoes and place in a bowl. Squeeze over the lemon juice and stir in the chopped basil. Season well.

3 To serve, place a slice of bread on each warmed plate and spoon over the tomato mixture. Garnish with basil leaves if desired.

Cook's note
Use wholemeal bread as a Healthy Extra and deduct 6 Sins per serving.

serves **4**

preparation
10 minutes
cooking time
about 3 minutes
✓ vegetarian

original

7 Sins

green

7 Sins

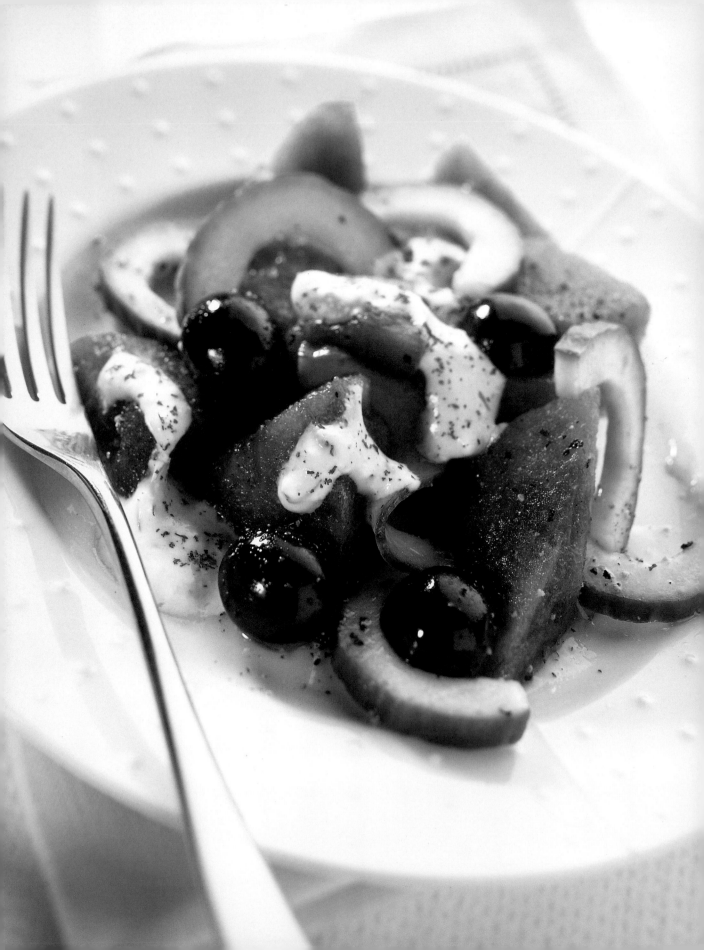

Watermelon salad with feta dressing

Bursting with colour and natural flavours, this wonderfully light, refreshing medley of watermelon, cucumber and grapes is the perfect starter for a steamy summer's day.

700g/1½lb watermelon

½ cucumber

40g/1½oz black or red seedless grapes

FOR THE DRESSING:

30g/1oz feta cheese, rinsed and dried

4 tbsp very low fat natural yogurt

1–2 tbsp chopped dill

salt and freshly ground black pepper

serves **4**

preparation

10 minutes,

plus chilling

✓ vegetarian

1 Cut the watermelon into large wedges, then slice the flesh away from the hard rind. Over a bowl to catch the juices, cut the watermelon into bite-sized chunks, picking out and discarding any seeds. Reserve the juice.

2 Halve the cucumber lengthways and scoop out the seeds, using a teaspoon. Cut the flesh into bite-sized slices or chunks.

3 Toss the watermelon, cucumber and grapes together in a large bowl. Cover and chill until ready to serve.

4 To make the dressing, crumble the feta cheese into a small bowl. Add the yogurt and reserved watermelon juice. Mash together until smooth. Stir in the chopped dill and season with salt and pepper to taste.

5 To serve, divide the chilled watermelon mixture between 4 salad plates and drizzle the feta and dill dressing on top.

original

1 Sin

green

1 Sin

Spinach and egg tartlets

Encasing a creamy, yet light spinach filling in paper-thin filo cases, these pretty tartlets make an impressive entertaining starter.

serves **4**

preparation
10 minutes

cooking time
15–20 minutes

✓ vegetarian

100g/3½oz chopped frozen spinach, thawed

2 large sheets of frozen filo pastry,
　　each 30g/1oz, thawed

1 large egg, beaten

3 tbsp very low fat natural fromage frais

2 tbsp finely grated Parmesan cheese

pinch of freshly grated nutmeg

salt and freshly ground black pepper

mixed salad leaves to serve

1　Preheat the oven to 200°C/Gas 6. Tip the spinach into a sieve and press well to remove excess water, then pat dry with kitchen paper. Set aside.

2　Lay the filo pastry sheets on top of one another and cut into 6 equal squares, to give you twelve in total. Line four 10cm/4in square non-stick Yorkshire pudding tins with a single pastry square. Brush with a little beaten egg and lay another filo square on top at a different angle. Brush again and top with the remaining pastry squares, to form 4 tartlet shells.

3　In a bowl, mix the remaining beaten egg with the fromage frais and 1 tbsp Parmesan. Stir in the spinach and sprinkle over the nutmeg. Season.

4　Carefully spoon the spinach filling into the tartlet shells and sprinkle over the remaining Parmesan. Bake in the preheated oven for 15–20 minutes or until the filling is set and the pastry is nicely browned. Serve immediately, accompanied by salad leaves.

original

3 Sins

green

3 Sins

Red pepper and potato frittata

This simple recipe transforms the humble egg into a delicious dish in a matter of minutes. Serve it as a starter or brunch.

serves **4**

preparation
10 minutes, plus standing

cooking time
15–20 minutes

✓ vegetarian

125g/4oz potato, peeled and cut into 1cm/½in dice

200g/7oz red pepper, cored and deseeded

Fry Light, for spraying

8 spring onions, thinly sliced

4 tbsp flat-leaf parsley, finely chopped

4 large eggs, beaten

salt and freshly ground black pepper

30g/1oz Parmesan cheese, freshly grated

sliced tomato salad to serve

1 Par-boil the potato in boiling salted water for 2–3 minutes. Drain and pat dry on kitchen paper. Cut the red pepper into 1cm/½in dice.

2 Spray a 20–23cm/8–9in non-stick frying pan (suitable for use under the grill) with Fry Light. Add the spring onions and stir-fry for 1–2 minutes. Add the diced red pepper and potato to the pan and stir-fry for a further 1–2 minutes.

3 Mix the chopped parsley into the beaten eggs, season and pour into the frying pan. Cook for 6–7 minutes or until the base is set. In the meantime, preheat the grill.

4 Sprinkle the Parmesan on top of the frittata and place under the grill for 4–5 minutes or until the frittata is well set and the top is golden brown. Leave to stand for 10 minutes, then carefully turn out the frittata on to a board and cut into quarters with a very sharp knife. Cut each quarter into 2 triangles and place 2 triangles on each plate. Serve with a tomato salad.

Cook's note
For a tasty alternative, substitute spinach for the red pepper.

original

2½ Sins

green

1½ Sins

Grilled vegetables with herb salsa

These delicious rosemary and thyme scented vegetables can be served hot, or at room temperature. Either way they are delectable drizzled with the fragrant, fresh-tasting herb salsa.

serves **4**

preparation

10 minutes

cooking time

8–10 minutes

✓ vegetarian

1 red pepper

1 yellow pepper

2 red onions, peeled

3 courgettes

12 cherry tomatoes

Fry Light, for spraying

2 garlic cloves, peeled and crushed

½ tsp crushed dried red chilli flakes (optional)

1 tbsp rosemary leaves, very finely chopped

1 tbsp thyme leaves

FOR THE HERB SALSA:

3 tbsp flat-leaf parsley, chopped

2 tbsp snipped chives

1 garlic clove, peeled and crushed

juice of 1 lemon

150ml/¼pt water

1 tbsp very low fat natural fromage frais

salt and freshly ground black pepper

TO GARNISH:

rosemary sprigs

1 First make the salsa. Place all the ingredients in a food processor and blend until fairly smooth, season to taste and set aside.

2 Halve, core and deseed the peppers and cut into bite-sized chunks. Cut the red onions into thin wedges. Thickly slice the courgettes. Put the vegetables and cherry tomatoes in a large bowl and lightly spray with Fry Light. Add the garlic, chilli flakes if using, rosemary and thyme. Season and toss to mix. Preheat the grill.

3 Spread the vegetables in a single layer on a foil-lined grill rack and grill under a high heat for 8–10 minutes, turning often, until they are just tender and slightly charred.

4 To serve, divide the vegetables between 4 serving plates and drizzle over the herb salsa. Garnish with rosemary sprigs.

original

Sin-free

green

Sin-free

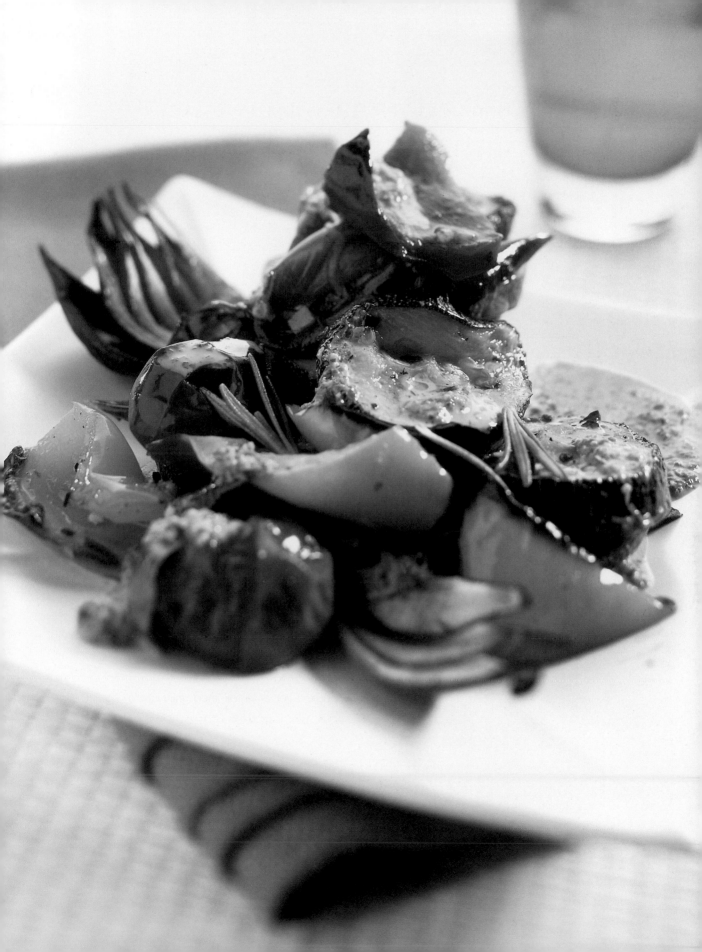

Stuffed portobello mushrooms

During baking, these meaty mushrooms release a wonderful Mediterranean aroma of garlic and rosemary.

serves **4**

preparation
10 minutes

cooking time
about 20 minutes

✓ vegetarian

4 large Portobello mushrooms, each
    8–10cm/3½–4in across

3 garlic cloves, peeled and crushed

4 spring onions, finely sliced

½ courgette, finely diced

1 red pepper, cored, deseeded and finely diced

1 tbsp chopped fresh rosemary leaves

juice of 1 lemon

1 tbsp water

salt and freshly ground black pepper

2 tbsp finely grated Parmesan cheese

1   Preheat the oven to 200°C/Gas 6. Remove the stalks from the mushrooms and place the mushroom caps, cup side up, on a non-stick baking tray. Chop the stalks and reserve.

2   Place the garlic, spring onions, courgette, red pepper, mushroom stalks, rosemary, lemon juice and water in a large non-stick frying pan. Cook, stirring, for 4–5 minutes or until the vegetables are slightly tender. Season.

3   Carefully spoon the vegetable filling into the mushroom caps and push down with the back of the spoon. Sprinkle over the Parmesan and bake in the hot oven for 15 minutes or until the cheese is golden. Serve immediately.

original

1 Sin

green

1 Sin

Italian-style mussels

Fresh mussels are cooked with red wine, tomatoes, fennel and herbs to create a sensational starter or light meal. Low in Sins, these mussels are cheap, delicious and quick to cook.

2 litres/3½pts fresh live mussels in their shells

3 shallots, peeled and finely chopped

2 garlic cloves, peeled and thinly sliced

½ fennel bulb, finely chopped

300ml/½ pt robust red wine

400g/14oz can chopped tomatoes

salt and freshly ground black pepper

3–4 tbsp flat-leaf parsley, finely chopped

serves **4**

preparation
10 minutes

cooking time
6–8 minutes

1 Scrub the mussels under cold running water and remove any barnacles or 'beards' with a sharp knife; discard any mussels that are open or cracked.

2 Place the shallots, garlic, fennel, wine and tomatoes in a large saucepan. Add seasoning and bring to the boil.

3 Add the mussels, cover the pan with a tight-fitting lid and cook over a high heat for 6–8 minutes, shaking the pan occasionally. Discard any mussels that do not open.

4 Stir in the chopped parsley, then ladle the mussels and liquor into 4 large serving bowls. Eat while still warm.

original

2½ Sins

green

7½ Sins

Gravadlax with cucumber and watercress cream

Gravadlax – smoked salmon flavoured with dill and white peppercorns – is a popular choice for a first course, and is conveniently sold pre-packed in supermarkets. Here it is enlivened with dilled cucumbers and a creamy watercress sauce to make a pretty, light starter.

serves **4**

preparation
15 minutes,
plus chilling

12 thin slices gravadlax or smoked salmon
FOR THE DILLED CUCUMBER:
1 large cucumber
2 tbsp chopped dill
1 tbsp white wine vinegar
salt

FOR THE WATERCRESS CREAM:
100g/3½oz Quark soft cheese
100g/3½oz very low fat natural fromage frais
85g/3oz watercress, trimmed
1 tsp creamed horseradish
freshly ground black pepper
TO GARNISH:
watercress sprigs
lemon or lime wedges

1 To prepare the cucumber, peel, halve lengthways, scoop out the seeds and slice thinly. Place in a bowl with the chopped dill and wine vinegar, season with salt and toss to mix well. Cover and chill until ready to serve.

2 To make the watercress cream, place the Quark and fromage frais in a bowl and stir until smooth. Finely chop the watercress, then stir into the Quark mixture with the horseradish. Season with salt and pepper to taste. Cover and chill until needed.

3 To assemble, divide the dilled cucumber between 4 plates and arrange 3 slices of gravadlax alongside. Place a dollop of watercress cream to the side, and garnish with watercress sprigs and lemon or lime wedges.

original

negligible

green

6 Sins

Cook's note
A terrific tool for finely chopping watercress and fresh herbs is a mezzeluna – an Italian curved chopping blade. Available from kitchen shops, it is very efficient and easy to use.

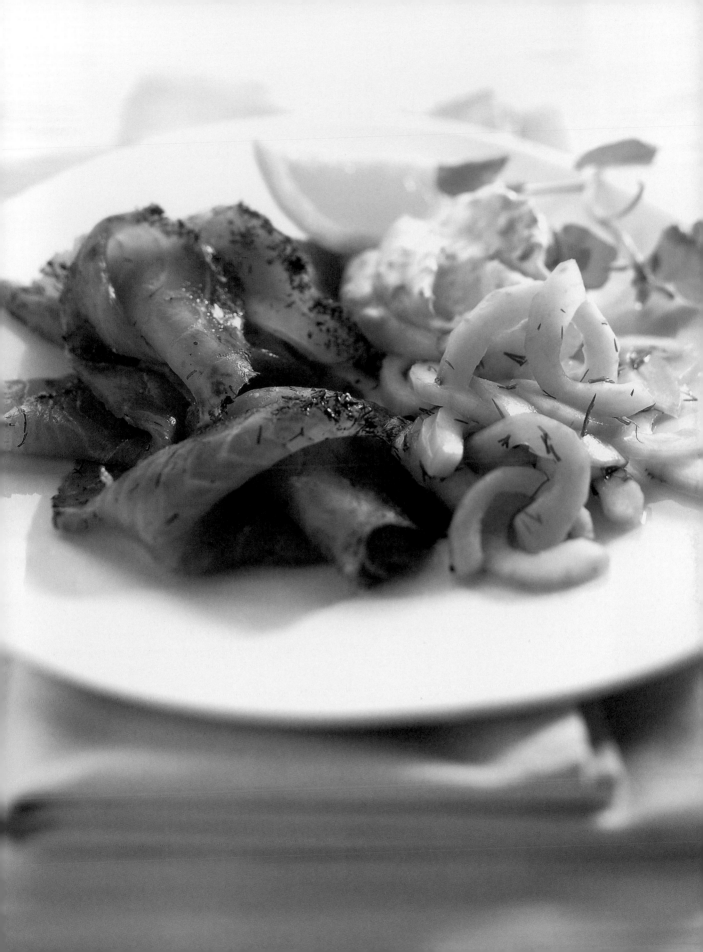

Grilled seafood skewers

These colourful, succulent skewers are delicious served as a starter with some wild rocket or other robust salad leaves. Monkfish is the ideal fish to use as it has a meaty texture that can withstand grilling.

serves **4**

preparation
10 minutes, plus marinating

cooking time
10–15 minutes

4 raw tiger prawns, peeled and deveined,
     but with the tail left on
450g/1lb monkfish or other firm white fish
     fillet, skinned
2 red onions, peeled
1 red pepper
1 green pepper

FOR THE MARINADE:
juice of 1 lemon
1 garlic clove, peeled and crushed
1 tsp crushed fennel seed
2 tbsp chopped dill
salt and freshly ground black pepper
TO SERVE:
rocket leaves
lemon wedges to garnish

1 First mix all the marinade ingredients together in a bowl, seasoning with salt and pepper to taste; set aside.

2 Place the prawns in a large bowl. Cut the fish into bite-sized chunks and add to the prawns. Pour the marinade over the fish and toss to coat evenly. Cover and leave to marinate in a cool place for 30 minutes.

3 Cut the red onions into wedges. Halve, core and deseed the peppers and cut into bite-sized chunks.

4 Preheat the grill. To assemble the skewers, thread the prawns, fish, onion wedges and pepper chunks alternately on to four long metal kebab skewers, or pre-soaked bamboo skewers. Brush them with any remaining marinade.

5 Place the skewers on the grill rack and grill for 10–15 minutes, turning occasionally, until the fish is just cooked through and the vegetables are just tender. Serve immediately, with rocket leaves and lemon wedges to garnish.

original

Sin-free

green

4½ Sins

Herbed tuna cream on lettuce leaves

Tuna is blended with fresh herbs and cottage cheese to make a delicious, quick pâté that requires no cooking. Served on sweet, crisp lettuce or other salad leaves, it makes an appetising starter.

200g/7oz canned tuna in water

2 tbsp chopped mixed herbs (dill, chervil and parsley)

juice of 1 lemon

200g/7oz very low fat natural cottage cheese, sieved

1 tsp grated horseradish or creamed horseradish

salt and freshly ground black pepper

2 Little Gem lettuces

1 Drain the tuna and pat dry with kitchen paper. Place in a blender with the chopped herbs, lemon juice, cottage cheese and horseradish. Season well and process until fairly smooth. Transfer to a bowl, cover and chill.

2 Separate the lettuce leaves, wash and dry well, using a salad spinner or clean tea towel.

3 To serve, arrange the lettuce leaves on 4 serving plates and spoon the tuna cream in the middle.

Cook's note

Try substituting canned red salmon, or fresh steamed trout or salmon, for the tuna. You can also flavour the pâté with different fresh herbs – a combination of fennel, parsley and chives works well. To further ring the changes, you might like to serve the pâté on bitter salad leaves, such as radicchio and endive.

serves **4**

preparation

10 minutes, plus chilling

original

negligible

green

2½ Sins

Spiced koftes with minted yogurt dip

Prepare your own chicken or turkey mince in a food processor for these delicious koftes. It only takes a few minutes and ensures you avoid any fat in pre-packed supermarket mince.

serves **4**

preparation

10 minutes,
plus chilling

cooking time

8–10 minutes

1 tbsp cumin seeds

85g/3oz very low fat natural yogurt

1 tbsp mild curry paste

4 spring onions, finely sliced

½ red pepper, deseeded and finely diced

2 tbsp chopped coriander leaves

salt and freshly ground black pepper

450g/1lb skinless, boneless chicken breast

Fry Light for spraying

FOR THE MINTED YOGURT DIP:

100g/3½oz very low fat natural fromage frais

60g/2oz very low fat natural yogurt

1 tbsp mint jelly

1 tbsp chopped fresh mint

TO SERVE:

mint leaves

lime wedges

1 Dry-fry the cumin seeds in a small pan over a low heat for 1–2 minutes, until the seeds release their aroma. Tip into a large bowl. Add the yogurt, curry paste, spring onions, red pepper and coriander; season and mix well.

2 Place the chicken in a food processor and blend until fairly smooth. Add to the yogurt mixture and mix well, using your fingers. Divide the mixture into 12 portions and shape each portion into a ball. Place on a non-stick baking tray and chill for 10 minutes.

3 Meanwhile, make the minted yogurt dip. Combine all the ingredients in a small bowl. Season with salt and pepper to taste, cover and set aside.

4 To cook, preheat the grill. Spray the koftes lightly with Fry Light and grill for 8–10 minutes, turning occasionally, until cooked through. Serve hot, garnished with mint leaves and lime wedges, and accompanied by the dip.

original

1 Sin

green

7 Sins

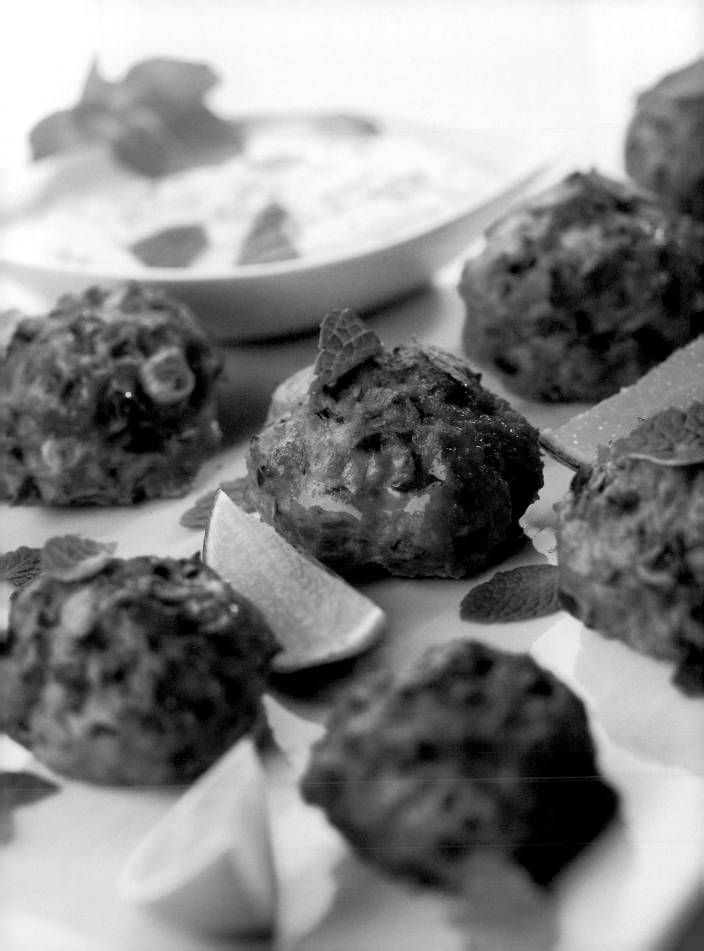

Parma ham with minted melon wedges

This instant, mouth-watering starter is wonderfully refreshing, especially on a warm summer evening. For optimum flavour, always use a fragrant, ripe melon. Pretty orange-fleshed Charentais is the perfect choice, but you can use a pale green Galia melon if you like.

serves **4**

preparation
10 minutes,
plus chilling

1 large, ripe Charentais melon

1 tbsp finely chopped mint leaves

1 tbsp lemon juice

8 thin slices lean Parma ham

freshly ground black pepper

mint sprigs to garnish

1 Halve the melon, then scoop out and discard the seeds, using a spoon. With a sharp knife, cut each half into 6 wedges. Cut away the skin from the melon; do this over a bowl to save any juices.

2 Carefully transfer the melon wedges and any juice to a large, shallow dish and sprinkle over the chopped mint and lemon juice. Chill until ready to serve.

3 To serve, arrange 3 wedges of melon on each serving plate and drizzle over the juices. Drape 2 Parma ham slices over each portion and season with pepper. Garnish with mint sprigs to serve.

Cook's note
You can vary this starter by grilling the Parma ham until crispy and serving it with cubes or balls of melon, rather than wedges.

original

Sin-free

green

4 Sins

Seared chicken livers on rocket leaves

This enticing starter of succulent, seared chicken livers is served hot on fresh, peppery rocket leaves. Allow time for the livers to marinate in the balsamic vinegar with herbs – you can then cook them in a matter of minutes. Ideally, they should be golden brown on the outside and still slightly pink in the centre, true French style.

450g/1lb chicken livers

4 tbsp balsamic vinegar

1 tbsp thyme leaves

1 tbsp chopped tarragon

salt and freshly ground black pepper

1 tbsp olive oil

60g/2oz rocket leaves

1 tbsp Parmesan cheese shavings

    to garnish (optional)

serves **4**

preparation

10 minutes, plus

marinating

cooking time

about 4–5 minutes

1 Carefully clean the chicken livers, removing any membrane, and pat dry with kitchen paper. Combine the balsamic vinegar and herbs in a large bowl. Add the chicken livers and turn to coat. Cover and leave to marinate in the fridge for at least 2 hours, but preferably overnight.

2 When ready to cook, drain the chicken livers, discarding the marinade. Season them well with salt and pepper. Heat the oil in a large non-stick frying pan. When hot, add the chicken livers and toss quickly in the pan until sealed and browned all over.

3 Divide the rocket between 4 serving plates and spoon the chicken livers on top. Garnish with Parmesan shavings if desired and serve at once.

original

2 Sins

green

8 Sins

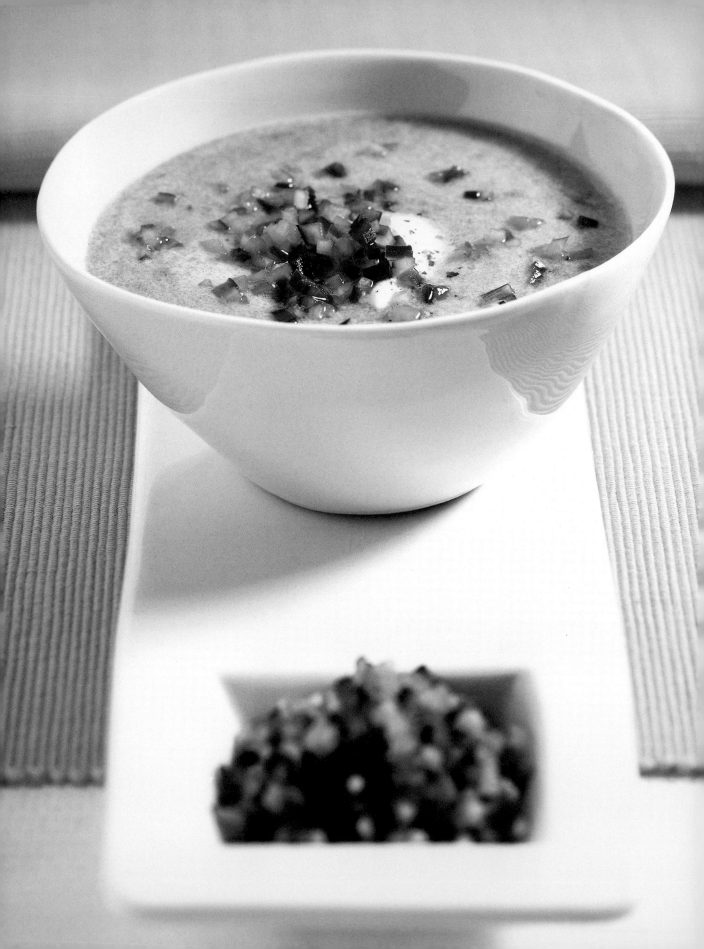

Creamy gazpacho

A perfect starter for a hot summer's day ... this classic chilled Spanish soup requires no cooking at all. Better still, you can make it a day in advance. Flavourful tomatoes are essential.

serves **4**

preparation
25 minutes,
plus chilling

✓ vegetarian

500g/1lb 2oz ripe plum or vine tomatoes

1 green pepper

1 small cucumber, peeled

3 spring onions, chopped

1 small red chilli, deseeded and finely
    chopped

2 garlic cloves, peeled and crushed

3 tbsp red wine vinegar

100g/3½oz very low fat natural yogurt

200ml/7fl oz cold water

salt and freshly ground black pepper

FOR THE GARNISH:

finely diced tomato, cucumber, yellow pepper
    and red onion

finely chopped coriander or parsley leaves

very low fat natural yogurt

1 Immerse the tomatoes in a bowl of boiling water for 30 seconds, then remove and peel away the skins. Halve, core and deseed the green pepper. Roughly chop the tomatoes, cucumber and green pepper and place in a food processor with the spring onions, chilli, garlic, wine vinegar, yogurt and water. Blend until smooth (see cook's note).

2 Pour the blended soup into a large bowl and season with salt and pepper to taste. Cover and chill in the refrigerator for several hours.

3 For the garnish, mix the diced vegetables with the herbs and place in small individual serving dishes. Put the yogurt in a separate bowl. To serve the gazpacho, ladle it into chilled bowls. Let guests help themselves to the garnishes.

Cook's note
If your food processor has a medium or small capacity, you will need to purée the soup in batches.

original

Sin-free

green

Sin-free

Chinese mushroom and tofu soup

A selection of tasty vegetables coupled with silken cubes of tofu makes this a nourishing soup to serve as a starter or light lunch.

serves **4**

preparation
10 minutes

cooking time
about 8 minutes

✓ vegetarian (see cook's note)

100g/3½oz baby pak choi or Chinese cabbage

85g/3oz carrots, peeled

6 spring onions

60g/2oz shiitake mushrooms

100g/3½oz tofu, drained

½ tsp finely grated fresh root ginger

1 garlic clove, peeled and crushed

600ml/1pt chicken stock, made with Bovril

2 tbsp dark soya sauce, or to taste

freshly ground black pepper

1 Finely shred the pak choi. Cut the carrots into thin matchsticks. Cut the spring onions into thin diagonal slices, and finely slice the mushrooms. Cut the tofu into 2–3cm/1in cubes.

2 Place the ginger, garlic and stock in a large saucepan and bring to the boil. Reduce the heat and simmer for 3–4 minutes.

3 Add the vegetables and tofu to the stock. Bring back to the boil, lower the heat and simmer for 2 minutes. Add the soya sauce and black pepper to taste. Ladle into warmed soup bowls and serve immediately.

Cook's note

For a vegetarian option, use vegetable rather than chicken stock. You can vary the vegetables, too. Try replacing the carrots with strips of cucumber, and use chestnut or enoki mushrooms in place of the shiitake. For a hot spicy note, add a thinly sliced small red chilli.

original

Sin-free

green

Sin-free

Corn and coriander chowder

Aromatic spices and fresh coriander perk up this hearty soup. Rich and satisfying, it is suitable to serve as a substantial starter or a light meal.

300g/10oz canned sweetcorn kernels, drained

200g/7oz potatoes, peeled

1 red pepper, cored and deseeded

Fry Light for spraying

1 large onion, peeled and finely chopped

3 garlic cloves, peeled and crushed

1 tsp ground cumin

1 tsp ground coriander

300ml/½pt skimmed milk

500ml/16fl oz chicken stock, made with Bovril

salt and freshly ground black pepper

2 tbsp very low fat natural fromage frais

3 tbsp chopped coriander leaves

1 Put half of the sweetcorn in a blender or food processor and work to a purée; set aside. Cut the potatoes and red pepper into 1cm/½in dice.

2 Spray a large saucepan with Fry Light and set over a low heat. Add the onion and garlic and cook for 4–5 minutes.

3 Stir in the ground cumin and coriander, the puréed and whole sweetcorn, milk, stock, potatoes and red pepper. Bring to the boil, reduce the heat and simmer for 10 minutes or until the potatoes are tender. Season with salt and pepper to taste.

4 Remove from the heat and stir in the fromage frais and chopped coriander. Serve immediately, in warmed soup bowls.

Cook's note

For a vegetarian soup, use vegetable rather than chicken stock.

serves **4**

preparation
10 minutes

cooking time
about 15 minutes

✓ vegetarian (see cook's note)

original

7 Sins

green

1½ Sins

Thai prawn and lemongrass soup

Fragrant, warm and comforting, this light, flavoursome soup is perfect for a cold evening.

serves **4**

preparation and **cooking time**

about 10 minutes

6 spring onions, finely shredded

2 fresh lemongrass stalks, very finely sliced

1 garlic clove, peeled and crushed

¼ tsp finely grated fresh root ginger

1 red chilli, deseeded and finely sliced (optional)

900ml/1½pts chicken stock, made with Bovril

60g/2oz shiitake mushrooms

60g/2oz mangetout

200g/7oz raw tiger prawns, peeled and deveined

1 tbsp dark soya sauce

2 tbsp chopped coriander leaves

1 Place the spring onions, lemongrass, garlic, ginger, chilli and chicken stock in a large saucepan, cover and bring to the boil.

2 Slice the mushrooms and mangetout thinly and add to the saucepan. Cook briskly for 3–4 minutes, then add the prawns and soya sauce. Cook for a further 2–3 minutes until the prawns turn pink. Take off the heat.

3 Stir in the chopped coriander and ladle the soup into warmed bowls. Serve straight away.

Cook's notes

● This soup is equally delicious made with chicken. Simply replace the prawns with 175g/6oz shredded cooked chicken breast (without skin), counting 4 Sins per serving on the Green choice.

● The vegetables can be varied, too. Try using thinly sliced carrots and pak choi in place of the mushrooms and mangetout.

original

Sin-free

green

2 Sins

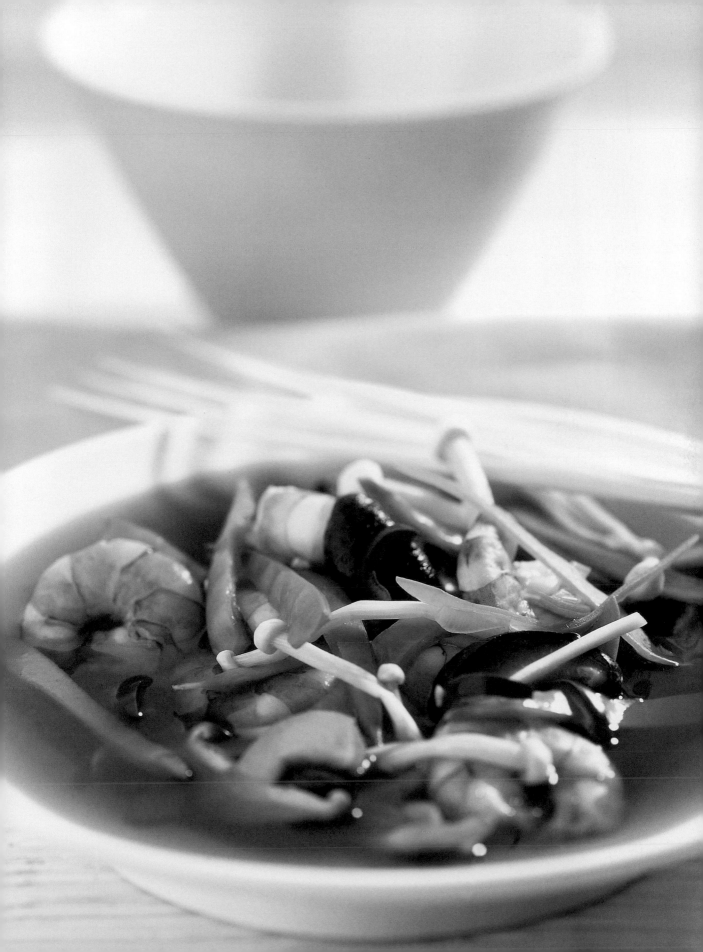

Chunky fish soup

A cross between a chowder and a fish stew, this delicious seafood soup is elegant enough to serve on special occasions.

serves **4**

preparation and **cooking time** about 15–20 minutes

2 garlic cloves, peeled and crushed

1 red onion, peeled and finely chopped

2 tbsp red wine vinegar

2–3 tsp granulated artificial sweetener

400ml/14fl oz vegetable stock

400g/14oz can chopped tomatoes with herbs

2 bay leaves

300g/10oz firm white fish (halibut or cod), skinned

300g/10oz fresh live mussels in their shells

200g/7oz prepared squid rings

250g/9oz raw tiger prawns, peeled and deveined

salt and freshly ground black pepper

3 tbsp chopped flat-leaf parsley

lemon wedges to serve

1 Put the garlic and onion in a large saucepan with the vinegar and sweetener. Mix well and heat gently for 2–3 minutes. Add the stock, chopped tomatoes and bay leaves, bring to the boil, cover and simmer for 5–6 minutes.

2 Meanwhile, cut the white fish into bite-sized chunks. Scrub the mussels under cold running water and remove the 'beards' and any barnacles with a knife; discard any with open or cracked shells. Add the fish and mussels to the tomato mixture and cook for 3–4 minutes.

3 Stir in the prepared squid and prawns and continue to cook, covered, for 2–3 minutes or until the squid is opaque and the prawns turn pink and are cooked through.

4 Remove from the heat, discard the bay leaves and any mussels that haven't opened. Season with salt and pepper to taste. Ladle into large, warmed soup plates or bowls. Sprinkle over the parsley and serve with lemon wedges.

original

negligible

green

7½ Sins

Italian chicken and tomato soup

This robust, satisfying winter soup, with its warm flavours of bacon, chicken and tomato, has a delicious citrus overtone.

1 onion, peeled and finely chopped

2 carrots, peeled and grated

2 rashers lean rindless bacon, finely chopped

2 skinless, boneless chicken breasts, each about 150g/5oz

600g/1¼lb canned chopped tomatoes

400ml/14fl oz chicken stock, made with Bovril

1 tbsp chopped rosemary leaves

finely grated zest and juice of ½ lemon

salt and freshly ground black pepper

1–2 tbsp chopped flat-leaf parsley to serve

1 Place the onion, carrots and bacon in a large non-stick saucepan and dry-fry the ingredients for 2–3 minutes.

2 Cut the chicken into thin strips and add to the pan with the chopped tomatoes, chicken stock, chopped rosemary, lemon zest and juice. Bring to the boil, stir, then cover and simmer on a medium heat for 15 minutes, stirring occasionally. Season to taste.

3 To serve, ladle the soup into warmed soup plates or bowls and sprinkle over the chopped parsley.

Cook's note

A little chopped lemon thyme is an excellent alternative to the lemon zest. You can, of course, use fresh rather than canned tomatoes for the soup, but will need to skin them first: place in a bowl of boiling water for about 30 seconds, then take out and peel away the skins.

serves **4**

preparation and **cooking time**
about 25 minutes

original

Sin-free

green

5 Sins

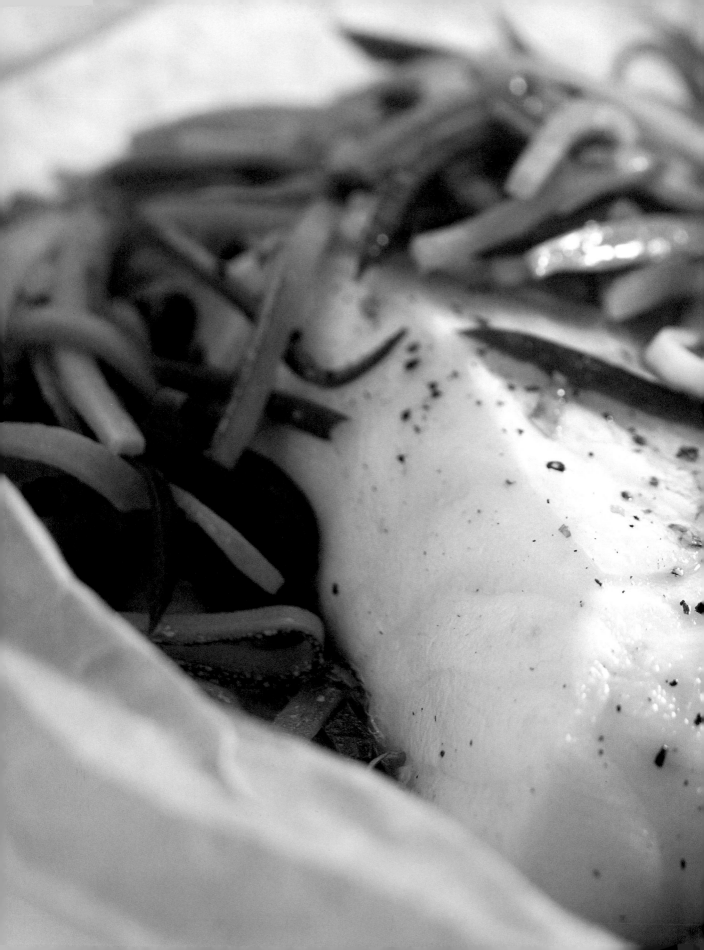

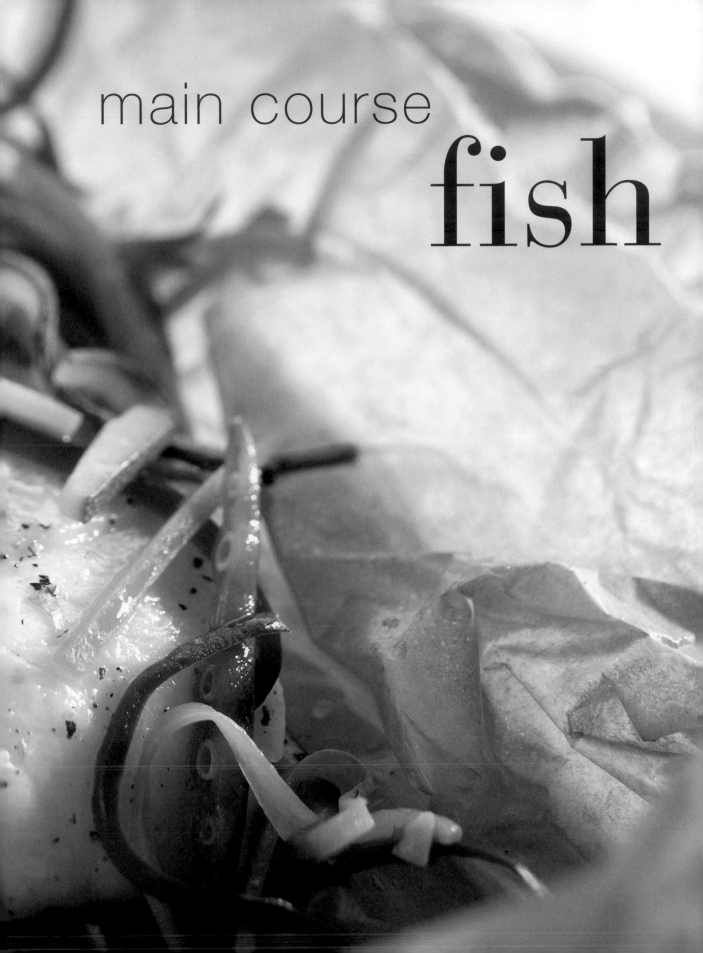

main course
fish

Baltimore fish cakes

The ultimate comfort food, these fish cakes are very low in Sins on an Original day. Use cod or halibut as an alternative to salmon if you like.

serves **4**

preparation
10 minutes,
plus chilling

cooking time
about 10–12
minutes

300g/10oz boiled, peeled potatoes

2 tbsp very low fat natural yogurt

1 tsp paprika

2 tbsp finely chopped flat-leaf parsley

2 tbsp finely chopped dill

4 spring onions, finely chopped

400g/14oz salmon fillet, skinned

½ beaten egg

salt and freshly ground black pepper

1 tbsp plain flour

Fry Light for spraying

1   Place the potatoes in a large bowl and mash until smooth. Stir in the yogurt, paprika, herbs and spring onions. Mix well.

2   Wash the salmon and pat dry with kitchen paper. Cook in a steamer over boiling water for 6–8 minutes or until just cooked.

3   Flake the salmon into the potato mixture, add the beaten egg and season well. Mix thoroughly, using your fingers. Cover and chill in the refrigerator for 30 minutes.

4   Divide the mixture into 8 portions and shape each one into a ball. Flatten each ball with your hands to form a 'cake' and lightly dust with the flour.

5   Spray a large, non-stick frying pan with Fry Light and place over a medium heat. Cook the fish cakes for 2–3 minutes on each side or until golden. Serve at once, with steamed spinach or another green vegetable.

original

3½ Sins

green

9½ Sins

Cook's note

If you have steamed a whole salmon (or a large piece) the day before and have some left over, this is the ideal recipe to use it up.

Spicy crab wedges

Easy and very quick to prepare, these tasty crab wedges are conveniently based on storecupboard ingredients. If you are feeling extravagant, use fresh white crabmeat...you will appreciate the difference in flavour and texture.

2 x 200g/7oz cans white crabmeat in brine

1 small red onion, peeled and finely chopped

1 green chilli, deseeded and finely chopped

2 tbsp chopped coriander leaves

salt and freshly ground black pepper

6 eggs

½ tsp Tabasco

2 tbsp Worcestershire sauce

Fry Light for spraying

mixed salad leaves to serve

serves **4**

preparation

10 minutes

cooking time

about 15 minutes

1 Drain the crabmeat and place in a large bowl with the onion, chilli and coriander. Season and set aside.

2 In a bowl, beat the eggs with the Tabasco, Worcestershire sauce, and salt and pepper.

3 Lightly spray a 23cm/9in non-stick frying pan with Fry Light and place over a medium heat. When the pan is hot, add the egg mixture and cook for 4–5 minutes, swirling the uncooked egg mixture around. Scatter the crab mixture over the surface.

4 Cover the frying pan, and cook gently for 8–10 minutes or until the base is golden brown and the mixture is set. Remove from the heat.

5 Leave to stand for a few minutes, then cut into wedges and serve with a crisp mixed salad.

original

Sin-free

green

3½ Sins

Moroccan spiced fish kebabs

Firm-textured monkfish is the perfect fish to use for these succulent kebabs, although raw tiger or king prawns can be used instead. Allow time for marinating, so that the spices can infuse the fish with their warm flavours.

serves **4**

preparation
10 minutes, plus marinating

cooking time
about 10 minutes

150g/5oz very low fat natural yogurt

1 garlic clove, peeled and crushed

1 tsp ground coriander

2 tsp ground cumin

½ tsp ground cinnamon

1 tsp freshly ground black pepper

1 tsp finely grated fresh root ginger

500g/1lb 2oz monkfish fillet, skinned

2 small red onions, peeled and quartered

8 baby plum or cherry tomatoes

TO SERVE:

shredded mint or parsley to garnish

lime wedges

1 Place the yogurt, garlic, coriander, cumin, cinnamon, pepper and ginger in a bowl. Stir to mix well.

2 Wash the monkfish and pat dry with kitchen paper, then cut into bite-sized chunks. Add to the yogurt mixture, turning to coat completely. Cover and leave to marinate in the fridge for 1–2 hours.

3 Preheat the grill. Remove the fish from the marinade and thread on to 8 metal or pre-soaked bamboo skewers, alternating them with the onion wedges and tomatoes. Brush with the remaining marinade.

4 Place the kebabs on the grill rack and cook under the grill for about 10 minutes, turning frequently, until the fish is cooked and the onions are tender. Serve immediately, sprinkled with shredded mint or parsley, and accompanied by lime wedges.

original

Sin-free

green

4 Sins

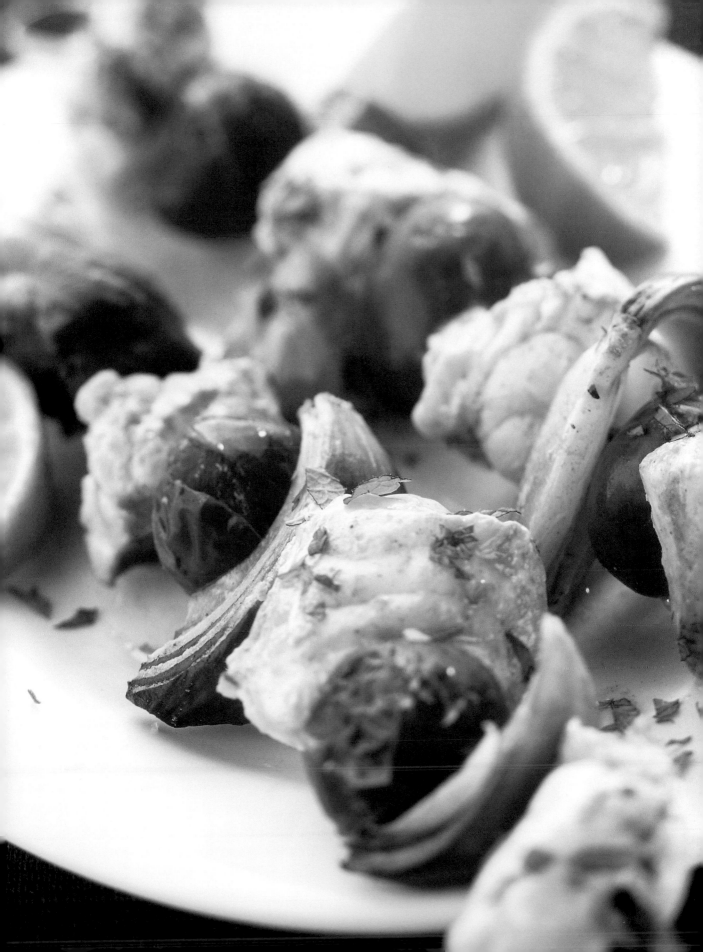

Creamy prawn curry

Juicy, large prawns and courgette form the basis for this aromatic curry, which is perfectly offset by crisp cooked cabbage, scented with cardamom and roasted cumin seeds.

serves **4**

preparation
10 minutes

cooking time
about 10 minutes

1 onion, peeled and finely chopped

1 garlic clove, peeled and crushed

1 tsp finely grated fresh root ginger

1 tsp ground cumin

1 tsp ground coriander

1 tsp paprika

200ml/7fl oz chicken stock, made with Bovril

1 large courgette

200ml/7fl oz passata

600g/1¼lb cooked, peeled tiger or king prawns

200g/7oz very low fat natural fromage frais

4 tbsp chopped coriander leaves

3 tbsp chopped mint leaves

salt and freshly ground black pepper

FOR THE CABBAGE:

½ green or Savoy cabbage, cored

seeds from 1 green cardamom pod, crushed

1 tsp roasted cumin seeds

TO GARNISH:

lime wedges

1 Put the onion, garlic, ginger, cumin, coriander, paprika and stock in a large saucepan, bring to the boil and simmer for 4–5 minutes.

2 Meanwhile, roughly chop the cabbage. Add to a pan of boiling water and cook for 5–6 minutes.

3 Cut the courgette into bite-sized pieces and add to the stock mixture with the passata. Bring back to the boil and simmer for a few minutes until the courgette and onion are tender. Stir in the prawns, fromage frais and chopped herbs. Heat through gently, then season and remove from the heat.

4 As soon as the cabbage is just cooked, drain it thoroughly. Toss with the cardamom and cumin, and season with salt and pepper to taste.

5 Serve the prawn curry straight away, garnished with lime wedges and accompanied by the cabbage.

original

Sin-free

green

7½ Sins

Prawn and chive omelette

As eggs are Sin-free and quick to cook, it makes sense to include them in your diet occasionally. This versatile omelette is an ideal choice if you are having supper alone.

2 large eggs

1 garlic clove, peeled and crushed

1 tbsp low fat natural fromage frais

1 tbsp finely snipped chives

salt and freshly ground black pepper

Fry Light for spraying

60g/2oz cooked peeled prawns, roughly chopped

serves 1

preparation
5 minutes

cooking time
4–5 minutes

1 Break the eggs into a large bowl and add the garlic, fromage frais, chives and seasoning. Beat lightly with a fork to combine; do not overbeat.

2 Place a 15cm/6in non-stick frying pan over a medium heat and spray the base lightly with Fry Light. When the pan is hot, pour in the egg mixture, tilting the pan to spread the mixture evenly over the base. Quickly stir the mixture with a fork then, as the egg begins to set, gently lift the edges of the omelette so that any liquid egg can flow underneath.

3 Scatter over the chopped prawns and cook until the underside of the omelette is set and golden and there is virtually no liquid egg mixture left.

4 Fold the omelette over and carefully slide it out of the pan on to a warm plate. Eat immediately, with a crisp green salad.

Cook's note

You can vary the herb flavouring and filling as you like ... the possibilities are endless. Try the following combinations: mushrooms and parsley; smoked salmon and dill; tomato, chilli and coriander.

original

Sin-free

green

3 Sins

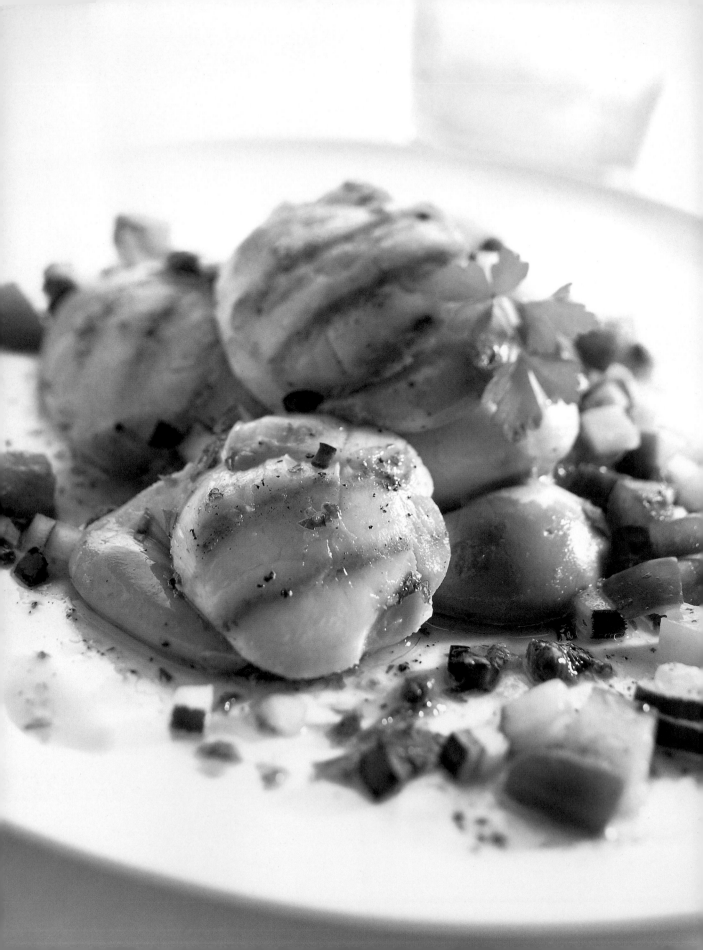

Griddled scallops with a herb dressing

A piquant dressing, made with a heady bunch of fresh herbs, capers and olives, accompanies succulent, seared, plump scallops. A fresh-tasting tomato and cucumber salad completes the picture.

500g/1lb 2oz shelled fresh scallops, with or
   without corals

Fry Light for spraying

salt and freshly ground black pepper

FOR THE HERB DRESSING:

2 tbsp chopped flat-leaf parsley

2 tbsp chopped mint leaves

1 tbsp chopped chives

finely grated zest of 1 lemon

2 tbsp white wine or tarragon vinegar

1 tbsp olive oil

1 tbsp capers, chopped

4 black olives, stoned and chopped

FOR THE SALAD:

3 ripe vine tomatoes, chopped

1 cucumber, chopped

1 small red onion, peeled and chopped

TO GARNISH:

flat-leaf parsley sprigs

serves 4

preparation
10 minutes

cooking time
about 6 minutes

1 First make the dressing. In a bowl, mix the herbs with the lemon zest, vinegar, oil, capers and olives. Season with salt and pepper and set aside. Place all the salad ingredients in a bowl and toss to mix. Set aside.

2 If necessary, remove the small tough, grey muscle from the side of each scallop, then rinse the scallops and pat dry with kitchen paper.

3 Heat a large, ridged griddle pan over a high heat. Lightly spray the scallops with Fry Light. When the pan is very hot, add the scallops and cook for 2–3 minutes on each side or until lightly browned, then remove.

4 Divide the salad between 4 large plates and arrange the scallops on top. Spoon over the dressing and serve immediately, garnished with parsley.

Cook's note

Fresh scallops are a wonderful treat, but do take care to avoid overcooking them, or they won't be juicy and tender.

original

1½ Sins

green

6 Sins

Griddled squid with Thai-style dressing

Quickly cooked on a ridged griddle pan, fresh squid is juicy and tender. Here it is tossed with a lettuce and cucumber salad, enhanced with a Thai-flavoured dressing, for a delicious light lunch or elegant main course.

serves **4**

preparation
10 minutes

cooking time
1–2 minutes

500g/1lb 2oz prepared fresh squid (pouches without head and tentacles)

FOR THE SALAD:
3 Little Gem lettuces
1 small cucumber
2 shallots, peeled and finely chopped
3 tbsp roughly chopped mint leaves

FOR THE DRESSING:
1 tbsp chopped fresh lemongrass
2 garlic cloves, peeled and crushed
2 tsp finely grated fresh root ginger
1 red chilli, deseeded and finely chopped
3 tbsp soya sauce
1 tbsp Thai fish sauce
1 tsp granulated artificial sweetener
juice of 1 lemon
1 tbsp chopped coriander leaves

1 Halve the prepared squid lengthways, rinse and pat dry. If the flat triangles are more than 10cm/4in long, cut them in half again. Using a sharp knife, score the inner surfaces in a lattice pattern, then set aside.

2 To prepare the salad, trim the lettuces, slice into fine strips and place in a large bowl. Peel the cucumber, halve lengthways and scoop out the seeds, using a teaspoon. Cut the cucumber into thin slices and add to the lettuce with the shallots and mint. Toss to mix.

3 To make the dressing, combine all the ingredients in a small bowl and stir to mix well. Pour the dressing over the salad.

4 Heat a ridged griddle pan over a high heat. When hot, add the squid and cook for 1–2 minutes or until the pieces have turned opaque and tightened into curls; do not overcook or they will become tough and rubbery. Add the squid to the salad, toss quickly and serve immediately.

original

Sin-free

green

4½ Sins

Herby salmon and prawn pie

Salmon. prawns and herbs transform this simple fish pie into something special. For a change. you might like to use a mixture of filleted fish. rather than all salmon. Serve the pie with steamed carrots and a green vegetable. such as courgettes or broccoli.

4 lean rindless back bacon rashers

4 eggs, beaten

175ml/6fl oz skimmed milk

115g/4oz very low fat natural yogurt

1 tbsp lemon juice

salt and freshly ground black pepper

400g/14oz salmon fillets, skinned

200g/7oz raw tiger prawns

30g/1oz reduced fat Cheddar cheese, grated

4 spring onions, finely sliced

2 tbsp chopped dill

2 tbsp chopped flat-leaf parsley

serves **4**

preparation

10 minutes

cooking time

20 minutes

1 Preheat the oven to 220°C/Gas 7. Roughly chop the bacon and dry-fry in a non-stick pan over a high heat for 2–3 minutes or until lightly browned. Transfer to a large bowl and set aside.

2 Place the eggs, milk, yogurt and lemon juice in a large bowl and whisk to combine. Season and set aside.

3 Rinse the salmon, pat dry and cut into bite-sized chunks. Peel and devein the prawns if necessary, then rinse and pat dry. Add the salmon and prawns to the bacon. Toss to mix well.

4 Spoon the salmon mixture into the base of a shallow ovenproof dish and sprinkle over the cheese, spring onions and chopped herbs.

5 Carefully pour the egg mixture over the top and bake in the hot oven for 20 minutes or until the filling is just set. Serve immediately, with carrots and a green vegetable.

original

2 Sins

green

14½ Sins

Salmon with tropical fruit salsa

Virtually Sin-free on an Original day, this colourful, healthy meal is perfect for easy entertaining. Experiment with different fruits to vary the salsa.

serves **4**

preparation
10 minutes

cooking time
15–20 minutes

4 salmon fillets, each about 200g/7oz,
    skinned
juice of 1 lime
2 tsp clear honey
1 tbsp light soya sauce
salt and freshly ground black pepper

FOR THE SALSA:
½ ripe mango, peeled
1 kiwi fruit, peeled
1 plum, halved and stoned
½ small pink grapefruit
1 tbsp mint leaves, finely chopped
TO GARNISH:
mint leaves

1 Preheat the oven to 180°C/Gas 4. Wash the salmon and pat dry with kitchen paper. Place each salmon fillet on a large square of baking parchment. Mix together the lime juice, honey and soya sauce and spoon over the fish. Season with pepper.

2 Bring the baking parchment up over the fish to form a parcel and fold the edges together to seal. Place on a baking sheet and bake for 15–20 minutes or until the fish is just cooked through.

3 Meanwhile, make the salsa. Finely dice the mango, kiwi fruit and plum. Peel the grapefruit, removing all white pith, then cut out the segments and finely dice them. Combine the fruits in a large bowl, add the mint and season with salt and pepper to taste. Toss to mix.

4 Unwrap the salmon and transfer to 4 warmed plates. Spoon over the salsa and serve immediately, garnished with mint leaves.

original

½ **Sin**

green

18 Sins

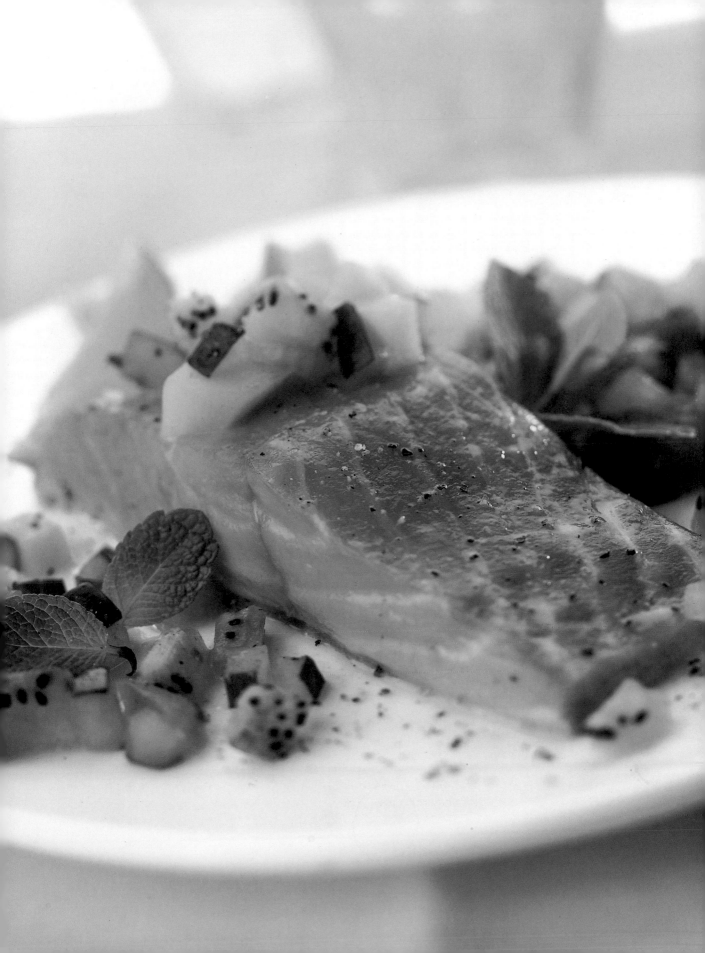

Steamed coconut and coriander salmon

The piquant flavours of chilli, fresh coriander, garlic, ginger and lemon permeate this fish as it steams – to delicious effect. Serve with boiled or steamed broccoli or cauliflower florets.

serves **4**

preparation
10 minutes

cooking time
12–14 minutes

4 salmon fillets, each about 200g/7oz, skinned

salt and freshly ground black pepper

FOR THE MARINADE:

2 tbsp reduced fat coconut milk

2 green chillies, deseeded and finely diced

2 tbsp chopped coriander leaves

2 garlic cloves, peeled and crushed

2 tsp finely grated fresh root ginger

juice of 1 lemon

100ml/3½fl oz hot water

TO GARNISH:

lemon wedges

coriander leaves

1 Line a steamer basket (that will hold the salmon in a single layer) with baking parchment. Make some tiny holes in the paper using a skewer, spacing them well apart. Rinse the salmon fillets and pat dry with kitchen paper.

2 Place all the marinade ingredients in a food processor and blend until fairly smooth. Transfer to a bowl.

3 Lay the salmon fillets in the lined steamer basket and spoon the marinade on top. Season with salt and pepper. Bring an 8cm/3in depth of water to the boil in the bottom of the steamer, then position the basket in the top. Cover and steam for 12–14 minutes or until the fish is just cooked through.

4 Carefully lift the fish from the steamer basket and place on warmed plates. Serve garnished with lemon wedges and coriander leaves.

original

½ **Sin**

green

18 Sins

Cook's notes

• Line the steamer basket with banana leaves rather than parchment, to impart a distinctive flavour. Look for them in quality greengrocers and ethnic food stores.

• If preferred, you can bake the fish in a covered dish in the oven rather than steam it. Preheat the oven to 180°C/Gas 4 and allow the same cooking time.

Chinese-style steamed fish

A whole sea bass, steamed the Chinese way – with ginger, garlic, soya sauce and sesame oil – looks spectacular, yet it is easy and hassle-free to prepare. A terrific centrepiece for a stylish dinner party.

1 sea bass, cleaned, about 1kg/2¼lb

salt

5cm/2in piece fresh root ginger, peeled and
   finely shredded

4 spring onions, finely shredded

4 garlic cloves, peeled and thinly sliced

3 tbsp soya sauce

1 tsp toasted sesame oil

freshly ground black pepper

serves **4**

preparation
10 minutes

cooking time
12–15 minutes

1 Rinse the sea bass and gently rub it with salt, inside and out. Set aside for 10 minutes. Mix the ginger, spring onions and garlic together and set aside.

2 Fill a steamer or wok with water to a level of 6–7cm/2–3in and bring to the boil. If using a wok, place a trivet under the base.

3 Rinse the salted fish under cold water and pat dry with kitchen paper. Place on a heatproof plate and sprinkle with the ginger mixture. Lower the plate into the steamer basket or on to the trivet in the wok, but don't let the plate touch the water. Cover, reduce the heat and steam for 12–15 minutes or until the fish is cooked through.

4 To serve, carefully lift the fish on to a serving platter. Mix together the soya sauce and sesame oil and pour over the fish. Season and serve immediately, with steamed broccoli.

Cook's note

If you do not have a wok or steamer large enough to accommodate a whole fish, you can steam the fish on a wire rack in a roasting tin. Lay the heatproof plate containing the fish on the rack and cover with foil, tucking it under the rim of the tin, to keep in the steam.

original

½ Sin

green

10½ Sins

Seared tuna with hot pepper sauce

Cooked in a flash, these juicy fish steaks – coupled with their piquant pepper sauce – make an ideal, midweek supper. Fresh tuna is now widely available from supermarket fresh fish counters as well as fishmongers; make sure you buy fish that is really fresh.

serves **4**

preparation

10 minutes

cooking time

about 15 minutes

4 fresh tuna steaks, each about 200g/7oz

Fry Light for spraying

sea salt and freshly ground black pepper

FOR THE SAUCE:

1 red onion, peeled and finely chopped

1 red pepper, cored, deseeded and finely
    chopped

1–2 red chillies, deseeded and finely
    chopped

1 celery stick, finely chopped

400g/14oz can chopped tomatoes

juice of ½ lemon

2 tsp Worcestershire sauce

½ tsp Tabasco sauce

TO SERVE:

100g/3½oz rocket leaves

chopped parsley to garnish

lemon wedges

1 Rinse the tuna and pat dry with kitchen paper. Lightly spray with Fry Light, season well and set aside.

2 To make the sauce, place the onion, red pepper, chilli, celery and tomatoes in a large, non-stick frying pan. Cook on a high heat for 8–10 minutes, stirring occasionally. Remove from the heat and stir in the lemon juice, Worcestershire and Tabasco sauces. Season to taste.

3 Meanwhile, heat a ridged griddle pan until very hot and place the fish on it. Cook for 2–3 minutes on each side; remove and keep warm.

4 Divide the rocket between 4 warmed plates. Place a tuna steak on each plate and spoon the sauce on top. Sprinkle with chopped parsley and serve with lemon wedges.

original

Sin-free

green

14 Sins

Cook's note
Swordfish steaks are a good alternative, if fresh tuna is not available.

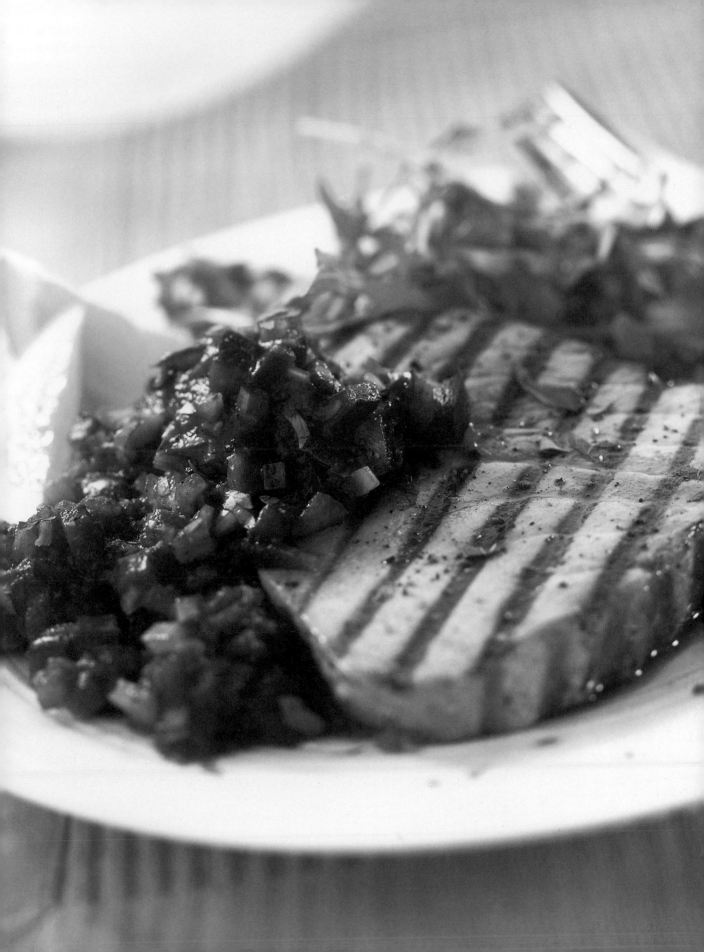

Charred chermoula mackerel with a citrus and olive salad

Exotic spices give pan-fried small, fresh mackerel a lively Moroccan flavour. A refreshing French bean, red pepper, olive and orange salad is the perfect complement.

serves **4**

preparation

15 minutes, plus marinating

cooking time

about 15 minutes

4 small mackerel, each about 300g/10oz, cleaned

1 tbsp reduced sugar apricot jam

juice of 1 lemon

2 tsp ground cumin

2 tsp ground coriander

2 tsp paprika

2 tbsp balsamic vinegar

salt and freshly ground black pepper

FOR THE SALAD:

100g/3½oz French beans, trimmed and halved

3 oranges

1 red pepper, cored, deseeded and thinly sliced

1 small red onion, peeled and cut into thin slivers

30g/1oz black olives in brine, drained

juice of 1 lemon

juice of 1 orange

1 Make 3–4 deep diagonal cuts on each side of the mackerel. Mix the jam, lemon juice, spices and vinegar together in a bowl; season. Rub the mixture all over the fish to coat evenly. Leave to marinate for 30 minutes to 1 hour.

2 Meanwhile make the salad. Blanch the French beans in boiling water for 2 minutes, then drain and refresh under cold running water. Cut the peel from the oranges, removing all white pith, then cut into segments. Place in a shallow salad bowl with the beans, red pepper, onion and olives.

3 Mix together the lemon juice and orange juice, season with salt and pepper and pour over the salad. Toss to mix well, cover and set aside.

4 Heat a large, non-stick frying pan until it is very hot. Place the fish in the pan and cook for 5–7 minutes on each side, until the surface is charred but the flesh is moist and cooked through. Serve immediately, with the salad.

original

1 Sin

green

23 Sins

Baked red mullet with pesto

The marriage of red mullet and pesto is a perfect one, and evokes flavours of the Mediterranean. Red mullet is available from good fishmongers and supermarket fresh fish counters. Just ask your fishmonger to scale and fillet the fish for you...with a smile, he should oblige!

2 lemons

8 red mullet fillets, each about 100g/3½oz

FOR THE PESTO:

3 garlic cloves, peeled and crushed

large handful of chopped basil leaves

3 tbsp freshly grated Parmesan cheese

1 tbsp extra virgin olive oil

juice of 1 lemon

100ml/3½fl oz water

salt and freshly ground black pepper

1 Preheat the oven to 200°C/Gas 6. Thinly slice the lemons and lay them over the base of an ovenproof dish, large enough to hold the red mullet fillets in a single layer. Wash the fish fillets and pat dry with kitchen paper. Lay them, skin side up, on the lemon slices.

2 To make the pesto, place the garlic, basil, Parmesan, olive oil, lemon juice and water in a food processor and process until fairly smooth. Season with salt and pepper to taste.

3 Spread the pesto over the fillets, using a small spoon and a brush. Bake in the hot oven for 12–15 minutes or until the fish is cooked through.

4 Using a fish slice, carefully lift 2 mullet fillets on to each serving plate. Serve with steamed greens or a mixed salad.

serves **4**

preparation

10 minutes

cooking time

12–15 minutes

original

2½ Sins

green

13½ Sins

Grilled trout with dill mayonnaise

Grilled fresh trout and blanched cucumber are enlivened by a creamy yogurt 'mayonnaise', flavoured with fragrant dill, piquant capers and gherkins. Salmon, mackerel and cod are suitable alternatives to trout.

serves **4**

preparation
10 minutes

cooking time
about 8–10 minutes

2 tsp mixed peppercorns

4 large trout fillets, each about 175g/6oz

Fry Light for spraying

salt

2 large cucumbers

FOR THE DILL 'MAYONNAISE':

5 tbsp very low fat natural yogurt

3 tbsp reduced calorie mayonnaise

1 garlic clove, peeled and crushed

1 tsp Dijon mustard

30g/1oz capers

30g/1oz gherkins

small bunch of dill, finely chopped

TO GARNISH:

dill sprigs

lemon wedges

1 Preheat the grill to high. Crush the peppercorns using a pestle and mortar or a rolling pin. Wash the trout fillets and pat dry with kitchen paper.

2 Lightly spray the grill rack with Fry Light and place the trout fillets on it, skin side down. Sprinkle with the peppercorns and season with salt. Grill for 5 minutes, then turn the fillets over and grill for 2–3 minutes.

3 While the fish is cooking, bring a large saucepan of water to the boil. Peel, halve and deseed the cucumbers, then cut into 3cm/1¼in dice. Add to the boiling water and blanch for 1–2 minutes. Drain and set aside.

4 For the mayonnaise, mix together the yogurt, mayonnaise, garlic, mustard, capers and gherkins, then stir in the chopped dill.

5 Serve the grilled trout immediately, scattered with dill sprigs and accompanied by the warm cucumber, lemon wedges and dill mayonnaise.

original

2 Sins

green

14 Sins

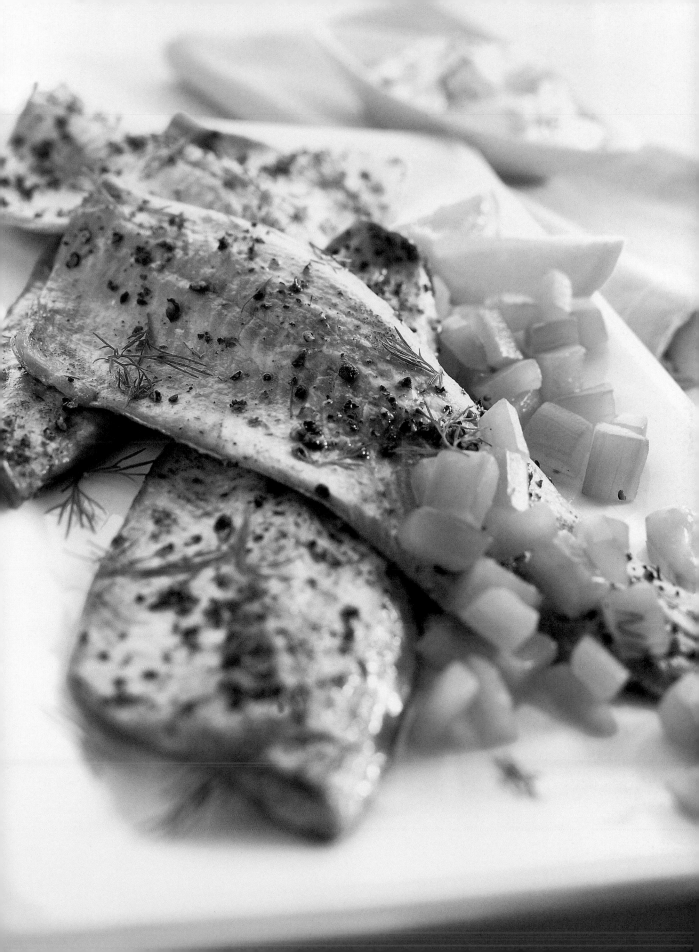

French fish stew

Sin-free on an Original day, this sustaining, tasty fish stew is ideal for quick and easy entertaining. Substitute cod for the monkfish if you wish.

serves **4**

preparation
10 minutes

cooking time
about 15 minutes

400g/14oz can chopped tomatoes

200ml/7fl oz chicken stock made with Bovril

2 tsp chopped oregano leaves

large pinch of saffron strands

3 garlic cloves, peeled and crushed

2 red peppers, cored, deseeded and
　　roughly chopped

4 baby leeks, cut into thick slices

1 courgette, cut into thick slices

350g/12oz monkfish tail fillet, skinned

salt and freshly ground black pepper

175g/6oz cooked, peeled tiger prawns

2 tbsp chopped flat-leaf parsley

1–2 tsp granulated artificial sweetener

1 Place the tomatoes, stock, oregano and saffron strands in a large saucepan and bring to the boil. Add the garlic, red peppers, leeks and courgette and cook briskly for 6–8 minutes.

2 Cut the monkfish into bite-sized chunks and add to the pan. Season and simmer gently for 3–4 minutes or until cooked through.

3 Stir in the prawns, chopped parsley and artificial sweetener. Stir gently, heat through and ladle into warmed large bowls. Serve straight away.

original

Sin-free

green

5½ Sins

Tandoori monkfish

Usually associated with chicken, this terrific recipe works well with firm white fish fillets, such as monkfish, halibut or Atlantic sea bass, too. Tandoori spice mixture, in a dry, powdered form, is available from most supermarkets and Asian greengrocers.

4 monkfish tail fillets, each about 150g/5oz

150g/5oz very low fat natural yogurt

3 garlic cloves, peeled and crushed

1 tsp finely grated fresh root ginger

1 tbsp tandoori spice mixture

juice of 1 lemon

salt and freshly ground black pepper

FOR THE SALAD:

1 small cucumber

1 small red onion, peeled

4 ripe plum tomatoes

2 tbsp chopped coriander leaves

1 tsp chopped mint leaves

juice of 1 lime

1 Wash the fish fillets and pat dry with kitchen paper. In a large bowl, mix the yogurt with the garlic, ginger, tandoori spice mixture and lemon juice. Season well.

2 Add the fish to the yogurt mixture and toss gently to coat. Cover and leave to marinate in the fridge for at least 3 hours, preferably overnight.

3 Preheat the oven to 200°C/Gas 6. Line a baking sheet with baking parchment. Lift the fish from the marinade and place on the lined baking sheet, in a single layer. Bake for 12–15 minutes or until cooked through.

4 While the fish is cooking, prepare the salad. Peel, halve and deseed the cucumber. Cut the cucumber, onion and tomatoes into 1 cm/½in dice and combine in a bowl. Add the herbs and lime juice, and season with salt and pepper to taste. Toss to mix well.

5 To serve, place the monkfish fillets on warmed serving plates and accompany with the salad.

serves **4**

preparation
10 minutes, plus marinating

cooking time
12–15 minutes

original

Sin-free

green

5 Sins

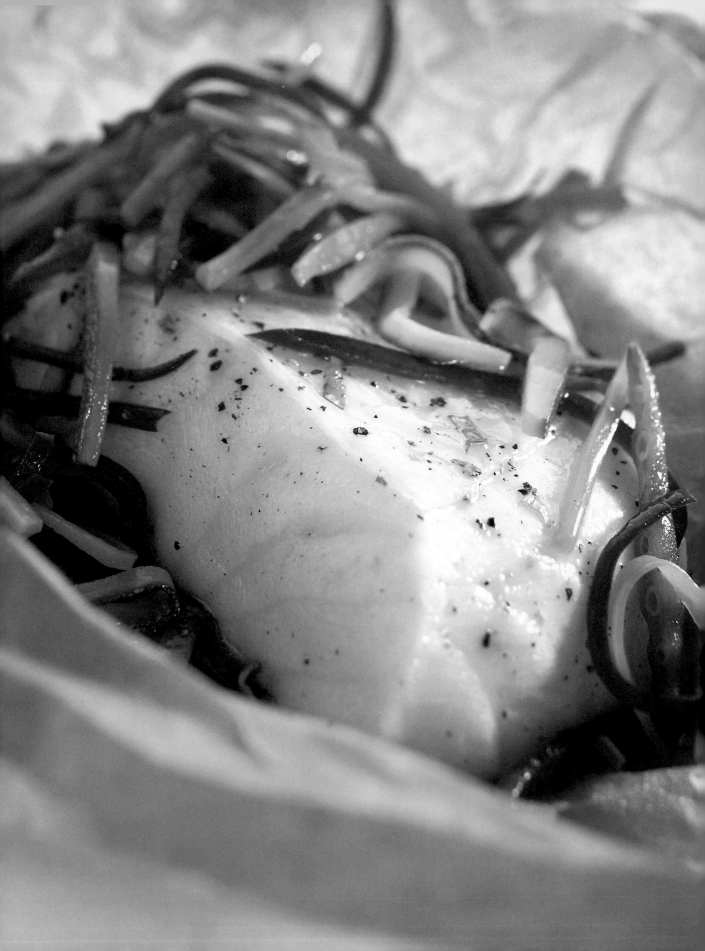

Cod and vegetable parcels

Cooking fish and vegetable julienne 'en papillote' is the perfect way to seal in their wonderful flavours and keep them deliciously moist. The parcels look impressive too, so this is a good choice for a main course if you are entertaining.

4 thick cod steaks or fillets, each about 175g/6oz

1 large carrot, peeled

½ courgette

1 red pepper, cored and deseeded

60g/2oz mangetout, trimmed

2 spring onions, trimmed

1 garlic clove, peeled and finely grated

juice of 1 lemon

1 tbsp chopped tarragon

1 tbsp olive oil

salt and freshly ground black pepper

1 Preheat the oven to 180°C/Gas 4. Wash the fish and pat dry with kitchen paper. Set aside.

2 Cut the carrot and courgette into thin matchsticks. Finely slice the red pepper and mangetout. Finely shred the spring onions. Place all the vegetables in a bowl and add the garlic, lemon juice, chopped tarragon and olive oil. Season with salt and pepper and toss to mix.

3 Cut 4 large pieces of baking parchment (generous enough to make roomy parcels for the fish). Put a portion of cod on each piece of parchment and top with a quarter of the vegetable mixture. Bring the edges of the paper up over the fish, fold them together and crimp to seal, making a parcel (without wrapping the fish too tightly).

4 Place the parcels on a baking sheet and bake in the hot oven for 15 minutes. Transfer the parcels to warmed plates and serve. Allow your guests to unwrap their parcels at the table.

serves **4**

preparation
15 minutes

cooking time
15 minutes

original

1½ Sins

green

7½ Sins

Baked haddock with steamed oriental greens

Soya sauce, orange and ginger bring the taste of the Orient to this dish. Pak choi, flavoured with sesame and lemon, is the ideal complement.

serves **4**

preparation
10 minutes, plus marinating

cooking time
about 15 minutes

4 haddock fillets, each about 125g/4oz

3 garlic cloves, peeled and finely grated

1 tbsp finely grated fresh root ginger

juice of 1 lemon

grated zest and juice of 1 orange

1 green chilli, deseeded and finely chopped

1 tsp clear honey

1 tbsp dark soya sauce

1 tbsp rice wine vinegar

1 star anise

FOR THE ORIENTAL GREENS:

6 small pak choi, halved lengthways

1 tsp sesame oil

1 tsp lemon juice

salt and freshly ground black pepper

1 Preheat the oven to 200°C/Gas 6. Wash the fish fillets and pat dry with kitchen paper. Mix the garlic, ginger, lemon juice and orange zest together in a small bowl. Rub this mixture all over the fish fillets and leave to marinate for 20–30 minutes.

2 Lay the fish fillets in a non-stick roasting tin, in a single layer. Mix together the orange juice, chilli, honey, soya sauce and vinegar. Pour this mixture around the fish and add the star anise. Cover the tin with foil and bake for 12–15 minutes.

3 Meanwhile, bring a 5cm/2in depth of water to the boil in a steamer. Place the pak choi in the steamer basket, cover and steam for 3–4 minutes or until just tender but still retaining a slight crunchiness.

4 Drain the pak choi, place in a bowl and drizzle with the sesame oil and lemon juice. Season and transfer to warmed plates. Top with the baked fish and pour over the pan juices.

Cook's note

Pak choi is a variety of Chinese greens, now widely available from larger supermarkets and greengrocers. Shredded green cabbage can be substituted.

original

1 Sin

green

5 Sins

Haddock and tomato roast

Succulent fillets of haddock are smeared with red pesto, scattered with fresh basil and roasted with tomatoes on the vine, to make an effortless main course. Serve with a steamed green vegetable, such as broccoli or courgettes.

4 haddock fillets, each about 200g/7oz, skinned

salt and freshly ground black pepper

2 tbsp red pesto

2 tbsp chopped basil leaves

20–24 cherry tomatoes on the vine

basil leaves to garnish

serves **4**

preparation

5 minutes

cooking time

16–20 minutes

1 Preheat the oven to 200°C/Gas 6. Line a roasting tin (large enough to hold the fish in a single layer) with baking parchment.

2 Wash the fish fillets and pat dry with kitchen paper. Place the fish in a single layer in the roasting tin. Season and carefully spread the red pesto sauce over each one. Scatter over the chopped basil.

3 Cover the roasting tin loosely with foil. Roast in the hot oven for 8–10 minutes, then remove the foil and arrange the tomatoes around the fish. Return to the oven and roast for a further 8–10 minutes, or until the fish is cooked through and the tomatoes are soft.

4 Transfer to warmed plates and serve immediately, garnished with basil leaves and accompanied by steamed broccoli or courgettes.

Cook's note

Pesto is an aromatic Italian sauce, traditionally made from fresh basil, pine nuts, garlic, olive oil and pecorino or Parmesan cheese – pounded together until smooth. Red pesto comprises the same ingredients, but derives its colour and flavour from the addition of sun-dried tomatoes. You can use green rather than red pesto for this recipe if you like.

original

1½ Sins

green

8½ Sins

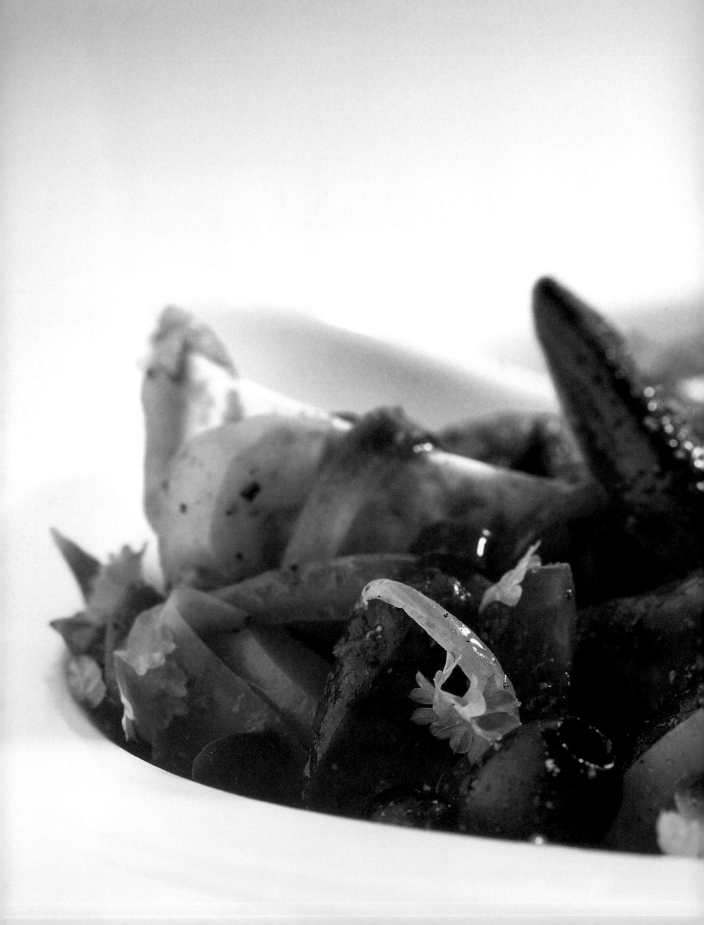

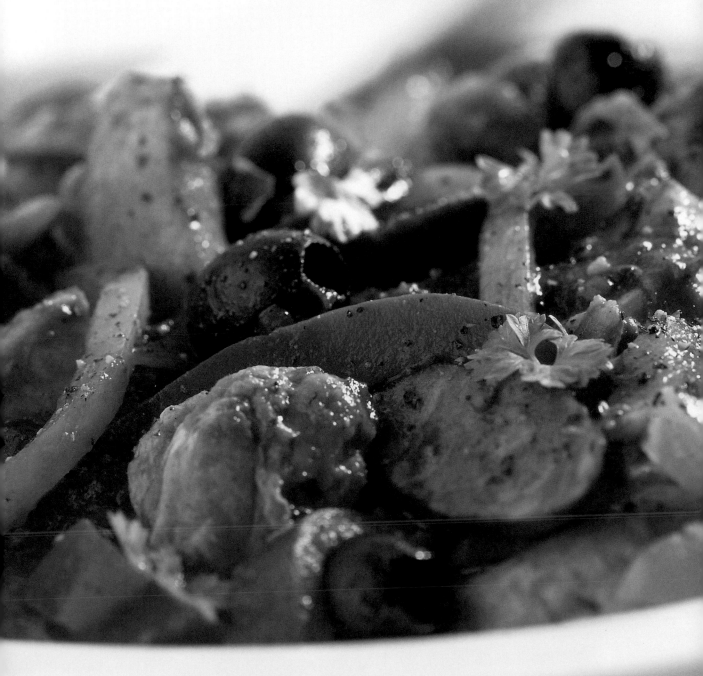

main course

meat

Chicken and Parma ham saltimbocca

Crisp, juicy and succulent, these chicken breasts are stuffed with ricotta, garlic and herbs and wrapped in smoky-flavoured Parma ham. For a pretty accompaniment, serve with steamed carrot and courgette julienne, or ribbons (see cook's note).

serves **4**

preparation
10 minutes

cooking time
20 minutes

4 skinless, boneless chicken breasts, each about 200g/7oz

4 slices lean Parma ham

FOR THE STUFFING:

150g/5oz ricotta cheese

3 garlic cloves, peeled and crushed

4 tbsp finely chopped mixed herbs (flat-leaf parsley, tarragon, rosemary and sage)

salt and freshly ground black pepper

TO GARNISH:

sage or flat-parsley sprigs

1 Preheat the oven to 220°C/Gas 7. To make the stuffing, mix the ricotta, garlic and herbs together in a bowl. Season with salt and pepper to taste.

2 Cut a deep slit along one side of each chicken breast to make a pocket. Divide the ricotta stuffing into 4 equal portions, spoon into the pockets and bring the edges together to enclose the filling.

3 Wrap a slice of Parma ham around each chicken breast, folding the ends underneath to seal in the filling. Carefully place the wrapped chicken breasts on a baking sheet lined with baking parchment.

4 Bake in the hot oven for 20 minutes, or until the chicken is cooked through. Serve immediately, garnished with sage or parsley.

original

2½ Sins

green

15 Sins

Cook's notes
• To prepare carrot and courgette ribbons, using a swivel vegetable peeler, pare along the length of the vegetable to shave off long ribbons. Briefly steam or blanch the vegetables separately in boiling water until cooked, but still slightly crisp.
• As an alternative to Parma ham, wrap the stuffed chicken breasts in blanched Savoy cabbage leaves, and count 13 Sins on the Green choice.

Parchment chicken

Cooking lemon and herb flavoured chicken 'en papillote' seals in the enticing aromas and delicious juices. Served with grilled tomatoes and steamed green beans, this dish makes an easy, impressive main course.

4 skinless, boneless chicken breasts, each
    about 200g/7oz
4 sage leaves, chopped
1 tbsp chopped tarragon leaves
finely grated zest and juice of 1 lemon

4 tsp reduced fat crème fraîche
salt and freshly ground black pepper
4 ripe plum or vine tomatoes
1 tbsp chopped basil

1 Preheat the oven to 200°C/Gas 6. Cut 4 large squares of baking parchment and place a chicken breast on each one. Sprinkle with the sage, tarragon and lemon zest. Squeeze over the lemon juice and spread a teaspoon of crème fraîche on top of each chicken breast. Season well with salt and pepper.

2 Bring the corners of the parchment up over the chicken and twist them together to form a tent-like parcel. Fold the edges of the paper together to seal and place the parcels on a large baking sheet. Cook in the oven for 15–20 minutes or until the chicken is cooked through.

3 Meanwhile, preheat the grill. Halve the tomatoes and grill them for 3–4 minutes or until softened. Sprinkle with the chopped basil and season well.

4 Unwrap the parchment and transfer the chicken breasts to warmed serving plates. Spoon over the juices and serve immediately, with the grilled tomatoes and steamed green beans.

Cook's note
Foil can be used instead of baking parchment, but you will need to spray it lightly with Fry Light to prevent the food from sticking to it.

serves **4**
preparation
10 minutes
cooking time
15–20 minutes

original
½ **Sin**

green
11 **Sins**

Coriander and mint grilled chicken skewers

These mouth-watering skewers are incredibly quick and easy to prepare and cook. Plan ahead if possible, so you have time to marinate the chicken in the spicy yogurt overnight...the flavours will permeate the chicken to delicious effect.

serves **4**

preparation
10 minutes, plus
marinating

cooking time
10–12 minutes

6 skinless, boneless chicken breasts, each
    about 200g/7oz
juice of 1 lemon
150g/5oz very low fat natural yogurt
1 tsp ground cumin
1 tsp ground coriander
1 tsp chilli powder

2 tsp clear honey
2 tbsp finely chopped coriander leaves
2 tbsp finely chopped mint leaves
salt and freshly ground black pepper
TO SERVE:
tiny mint leaves to garnish
lemon wedges

1 Cut the skinless chicken breasts into large, bite-sized cubes and place them in a large bowl.

2 Put the lemon juice, yogurt, ground spices, honey and chopped herbs in a blender or food processor and blend until fairly smooth. Season and pour this mixture over the chicken. Toss to coat evenly. Cover and set aside to marinate for 30 minutes, or preferably leave in the refrigerator overnight.

3 Preheat the grill. Thread the chicken pieces on to 8 metal skewers or pre-soaked bamboo skewers. Place on the grill rack and grill for 10–12 minutes, turning frequently until the chicken is cooked through.

4 Place the skewers on warmed plates and scatter with tiny mint leaves. Serve immediately, with lemon wedges and a mixed leaf salad.

Cook's note
Cubed boneless turkey steaks could be used as an alternative to the chicken.

original

½ **Sin**

green

16 Sins

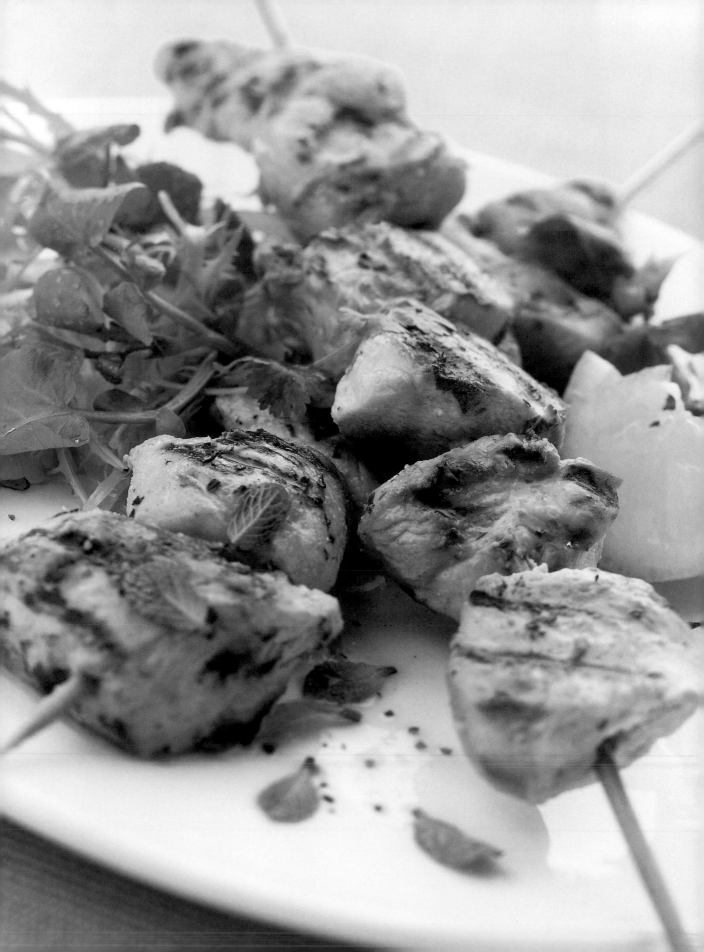

Chargrilled Caribbean chicken

Succulent drumsticks with a crisp, Caribbean 'jerk seasoning' coating are popular in Jamaica. Here they are grilled, but you can barbecue them in summer, or bake them in the oven if you prefer. Team with low fat yogurt and a crisp green salad for a satisfying main course.

serves **4**

preparation
10 minutes, plus marinating

cooking time
15–20 minutes

8 plump chicken drumsticks, each about
　　200g/7oz
FOR THE 'JERK' MARINADE:
3–4 allspice berries
1 tsp freshly grated nutmeg
1 tsp ground cinnamon
pinch of ground cloves
½ small red onion, peeled and finely grated

4–5 spring onions, finely sliced
1 red chilli, deseeded and finely chopped
finely grated zest and juice of 1 large lime
salt and freshly ground black pepper
TO SERVE:
very low fat natural yogurt
lime wedges

1　For the marinade, put the allspice berries in a small, dry, non-stick frying pan and place on a medium heat for 3–4 minutes, shaking the pan frequently, until the berries give off an aroma. Remove from the heat and place in a large mortar. Add the nutmeg, cinnamon and cloves, and grind with the pestle to a powder.

2　Add the red onion, spring onions, chilli, lime zest and juice, salt and pepper. Pound the mixture to a thick paste.

3　Slash the chicken drumsticks several times with a sharp knife and rub the 'jerk' marinade all over them. Place in a shallow non-metal dish, cover and marinate in the refrigerator for at least 1 hour, or up to 24 hours.

4　When ready to cook, preheat the grill to high. Place the drumsticks on the grill rack and cook under the grill for 15–20 minutes, turning occasionally, until cooked through. To test whether the chicken is cooked, insert a thin metal skewer or knife tip into the thickest part and check that the juices run clear.

5　Serve the drumsticks hot, with very low fat yogurt and lime wedges. Accompany with a crisp green salad.

original

Sin-free

green

12 Sins

Japanese-style chicken with vegetables

Marinate plump chicken breasts with Japanese flavours of soya sauce, ginger, sweet rice wine and honey, then grill to perfection and serve with a medley of oriental-style vegetables.

4 skinless, boneless chicken breasts, each about 200g/7oz

FOR THE MARINADE:

5 tbsp light soya sauce

2 tbsp sweet rice wine, or sweet sherry

1 tbsp clear honey

2 garlic cloves, peeled and finely grated

1 tsp finely grated fresh root ginger

finely grated zest and juice of 1 satsuma or small orange

FOR THE VEGETABLES:

Fry Light for spraying

4 spring onions, finely sliced

1 red chilli, deseeded and finely chopped

1 garlic clove, peeled and crushed

200g/7oz broccoli, cut into small florets

400g/14oz shiitake or chestnut mushrooms, finely sliced

1 tbsp dark soya sauce

salt and freshly ground black pepper

serves **4**

preparation

10 minutes, plus marinating

cooking time

about 12–15 minutes

1 Make 4–5 deep slashes in each chicken breast with a sharp knife, then place in a single layer in a shallow, non-metal dish.

2 Mix the marinade ingredients together in a bowl, then pour over the chicken and turn to coat. Cover and leave to marinate in the fridge for at least 1 hour, preferably overnight, turning occasionally.

3 To cook, preheat the grill to high. Place the chicken on a grill rack and grill for about 6–7 minutes on each side, brushing frequently with the marinade.

4 Meanwhile, heat a large, non-stick frying pan over a high heat and spray lightly with Fry Light. Add the spring onions, chilli and garlic and stir-fry for 2–3 minutes. Add the broccoli and mushrooms and stir-fry for 4–5 minutes or until the broccoli is just tender, but still has a bite. Add the soya sauce and seasoning.

5 To serve, place the chicken breasts on warmed serving plates and spoon over the juices. Accompany with the oriental vegetables.

original

1 Sin

green

11½ Sins

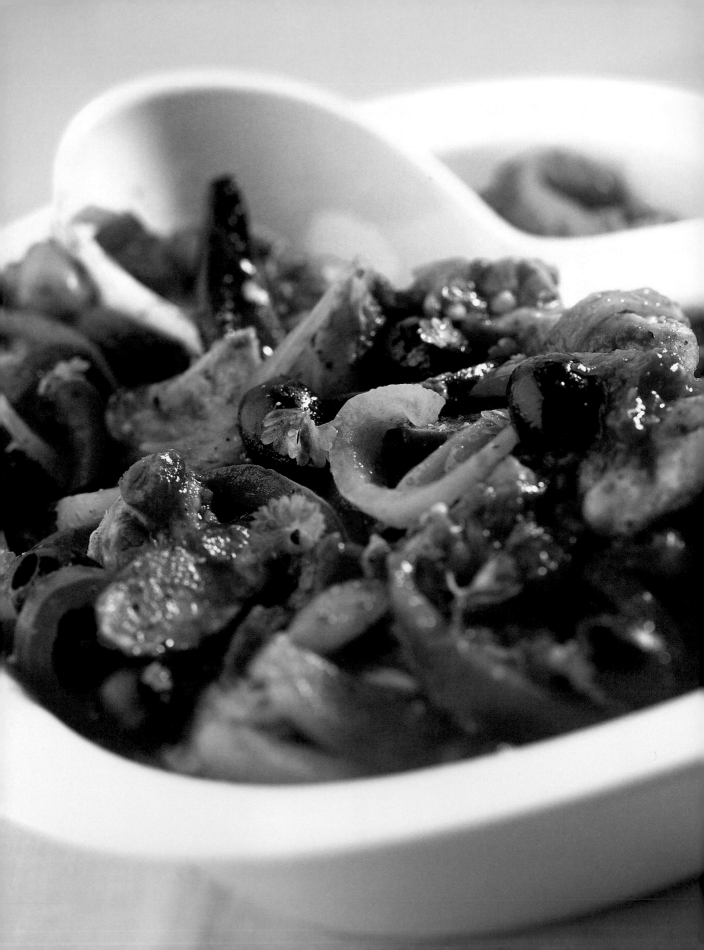

Spanish-style chicken

Sweet red and yellow peppers, spicy chorizo, dark olives and juicy, red tomatoes bring the flavours and colours of the Mediterranean to tender chicken, for an easy, one-pot family meal.

serves **4**

preparation
10 minutes

cooking time
about 20 minutes

8 boneless, skinless chicken thighs, about 500g/1lb 2oz in total

Fry Light for spraying

1 red onion, peeled and thinly sliced

2 garlic cloves, peeled and crushed

1 large red pepper, cored, deseeded and sliced

1 large yellow pepper, cored, deseeded and sliced

400g/14oz can chopped tomatoes with herbs

150ml/¼pt chicken stock, made with Bovril

1 tbsp sweet paprika

60g/2oz chorizo sausage, thickly sliced

12–15 black olives, pitted

salt and freshly ground black pepper

roughly torn parsley, to garnish

1 Cut the chicken into bite-sized chunks. Lightly spray a large non-stick frying pan with Fry Light and place over a high heat. Add the chicken and fry, turning, until sealed and golden.

2 Add the onion and garlic and cook, stirring, for 1 minute, then add the peppers. Stir and cook for a further 3–4 minutes until slightly softened.

3 Stir in the tomatoes, stock and paprika and bring to the boil. Add the chorizo to the frying pan and simmer for 15 minutes or until the chicken is cooked. Stir in the olives and season well.

4 Transfer to a warmed serving dish. Scatter with the parsley and serve immediately, accompanied by a green salad.

Cook's note

You can substitute garlic sausage for the chorizo if you like.

original

2 Sins

green

9½ Sins

Herby mushroom and cheese turkey rolls

Turkey breast steaks are rolled around a low fat soft cheese stuffing – flavoured with aromatic herbs, garlic and mushrooms – then cooked until tender. For optimum effect, serve sliced, with a selection of steamed or boiled vegetables.

serves **4**

preparation
10 minutes

cooking time
about 15 minutes

4 skinless, boneless turkey breast steaks, each about 200g/7oz
200g/7oz Quark skimmed milk soft cheese
60g/2oz mushrooms, very finely chopped
2 garlic cloves, peeled and finely grated
2 tbsp chopped mixed herbs (parsley, sage, rosemary and thyme)
salt and freshly ground black pepper

1 Place the turkey breast steaks between two sheets of cling film or greaseproof paper on your work surface and flatten them out until about 1.5cm/⅝in thin, using a meat mallet or rolling pin. Set aside.

2 Place the Quark in a bowl and stir until smooth. Add the mushrooms, garlic and chopped herbs. Season generously and mix well.

3 Uncover the flattened turkey steaks, spread with the cheese mixture and carefully roll each one up into a sausage shape. Wrap each turkey roll tightly in foil and twist the ends to seal the parcels.

4 One-third fill a large saucepan with water and bring to the boil. Add the foil parcels and simmer gently for 12–15 minutes, then remove.

5 Carefully unwrap the parcels and thickly slice the turkey. Serve immediately, with a selection of boiled or steamed vegetables.

original

Sin-free

green

10½ Sins

Creamy turkey and mushroom ragoût

Tender strips of turkey are cooked gently with spring onions and mushrooms, then served in a creamy sauce spiked with grainy mustard. Serve with swede or celeriac mash (see page 114) for a satisfying meal.

500g/1lb 2oz turkey breast fillets

Fry Light for spraying

1 garlic clove, peeled and finely chopped

6 spring onions, finely sliced

200g/7oz button mushrooms, finely sliced

salt and freshly ground black pepper

150ml/¼pt chicken stock, made with Bovril

4 tbsp reduced fat crème fraîche

1 tbsp wholegrain mustard

1 tsp cornflour, mixed with 1 tbsp cold water

chopped parsley to garnish

1 Cut the turkey into thin strips. Spray a large non-stick pan with Fry Light, add the turkey strips and cook over a moderate heat for 4–5 minutes, turning occasionally, until golden.

2 Add the garlic, spring onions and mushrooms to the pan. Season with salt and pepper and cook for 3–4 minutes.

3 Pour in the stock and bring to the boil, then stir in the crème fraîche and mustard. Bring back to the boil, stir in the blended cornflour and simmer gently, stirring, for 4–5 minutes until thickened and smooth.

4 Ladle the ragoût into warmed deep plates, sprinkle with chopped parsley and serve straight away.

Cook's note

You can, of course, use chicken breast fillets rather than turkey if you prefer.

serves **4**

preparation
10 minutes
cooking time
about 15 minutes

original

2 Sins

green

9 Sins

Grilled gammon steaks and tomatoes with herb mash

Juicy gammon steaks are grilled with flavourful vine tomatoes and served with a tempting creamy mash of swede, spring onions and herbs for an excellent casual supper.

serves **4**

preparation
10 minutes

cooking time
about 15 minutes

4 lean smoked gammon steaks, each about
200g/7oz
16–20 midi plum tomatoes on the vine,
halved
salt and freshly ground black pepper
FOR THE MASH:
500g/1lb 2oz swede

6 spring onions, finely chopped
3 tbsp chopped fresh parsley
2 tbsp chopped fresh basil
100g/3½oz very low fat natural fromage frais
salt and freshly ground black pepper
TO GARNISH:
roughly torn basil leaves

1 First prepare the mash. Cut the peel from the swede and roughly chop the flesh into small chunks. Cook in boiling water for 12–15 minutes until tender.

2 Meanwhile, mix the spring onions, chopped herbs and fromage frais together in a bowl.

3 Preheat the grill. Lay the gammon steaks on a foil-lined large grill pan and place the tomatoes around them. Season and grill for 6–8 minutes, turning the steaks halfway through grilling.

4 When the swede is cooked, drain it thoroughly, then mash. Add the fromage frais mixture and combine well. Season and keep warm.

5 To serve, place the gammon steaks on warmed plates with the grilled tomatoes. Spoon the herb mash alongside and serve immediately, garnished with basil.

original

Sin-free

green

14 Sins

Cook's notes
• Midi plum tomatoes are larger than baby ones, but smaller than the standard variety. If unobtainable, use 8 ordinary plum tomatoes, halved, instead.
• To vary the flavour of the mash, try using celeriac in place of swede.

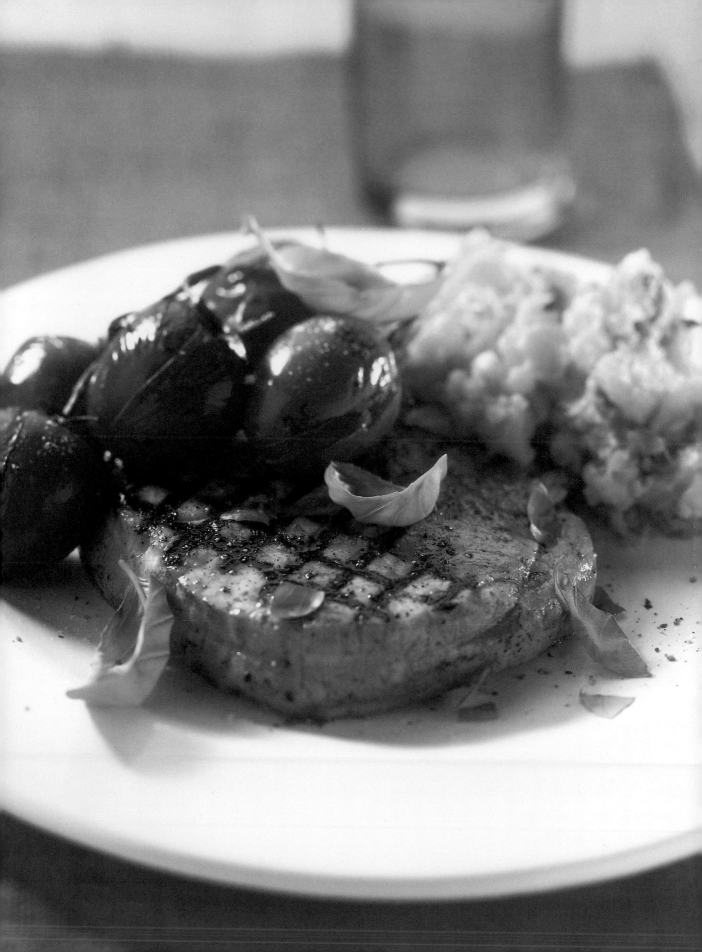

Honey, soy and ginger duck breasts

A piquant sauce, flavoured with raspberry vinegar, ginger, soya sauce and honey enhances pan-fried skinless duck breast…to excellent effect. The duck is sliced and served on a bed of wilted leeks to further whet the appetite.

serves **4**

preparation

10 minutes

cooking time

about 20 minutes

4 boneless duck breasts, each about 200g/7oz, skinned and trimmed of visible fat

2 medium leeks, trimmed

3 tbsp raspberry wine vinegar

20g/¾oz fresh root ginger, peeled and cut into very thin strips

2 tbsp dark soya sauce

500ml/16fl oz chicken stock made with Bovril

1 tbsp clear honey

1 tsp arrowroot, mixed with 3 tbsp cold water

Fry Light for spraying

salt and freshly ground black pepper

1 Preheat the oven to low. Heat a large non-stick frying pan over a moderate heat and dry-fry the duck breasts on each side for about 5–6 minutes.

2 Meanwhile, halve the leeks lengthways, rinse well, then cut into matchstick-sized strips and set aside.

3 Transfer the cooked duck to a plate and put in the oven to keep warm. Add the vinegar to the frying pan and bring to the boil. Add the ginger, soya sauce, stock and honey and return to the boil. Reduce the heat, stir in the arrowroot mixture and cook gently, stirring, for 5–6 minutes or until the sauce has thickened slightly.

4 Meanwhile spray a non-stick frying pan with Fry Light and add the leeks. Cook over a moderate heat for 3–4 minutes until just tender. Season and set aside.

5 Return the duck to the ginger sauce and reheat for 1–2 minutes. Check the seasoning. Remove the duck breasts from the sauce and slice diagonally. Divide the leeks between warmed plates, and arrange the sliced duck breasts on top. Spoon over the sauce and serve immediately.

original

½ Sin

green

14½ Sins

Peppered venison steaks with a fruity mash

Lean venison steaks are spiked with a peppery coating flavoured with juniper, then pan-fried and served with a tasty mash of apple, leek and swede.

2 tbsp mixed peppercorns

2–3 juniper berries

4 lean venison steaks, each about 175g/6oz

Fry Light for spraying

FOR THE MASH:

500g/1lb 2oz swede

2 medium leeks

2 dessert apples

salt and freshly ground black pepper

serves **4**

preparation

10 minutes

cooking time

about 20 minutes

1 Crush the peppercorns and juniper berries coarsely, using a pestle and mortar or rolling pin. Lightly coat the venison steaks with the peppercorn mixture, pressing it firmly into the flesh. Set aside.

2 To prepare the mash, cut the peel from the swede and roughly chop the flesh into small chunks. Cook in boiling water for 12–15 minutes until tender.

3 Meanwhile, halve the leeks lengthways, rinse and slice very finely. Add to a pan of boiling water and boil for 2–3 minutes or until tender. Drain and set aside.

4 Peel, core and finely chop the apples. Heat a non-stick pan on a medium heat and spray with Fry Light. Add the apples and cook for 2–3 minutes or until soft. When the swede is cooked, drain it thoroughly, then mash. Fold in the leeks and apples, then season, cover and keep warm.

5 Heat a ridged griddle pan over a high heat. Lightly spray the venison steaks with Fry Light. When the pan is hot, add the steaks and cook for 2 minutes on each side for medium-rare, or up to 4 minutes if you prefer venison medium or well done. Season and serve on warmed plates, accompanied by the mash.

original

1½ Sins

green

10½ Sins

Chive and ginger pork stir-fry

The flavours of France and the Orient combine in this intriguing and colourful stir-fry. Strips of chicken can be used as an alternative to pork if you like.

serves **4**

preparation
10 minutes

cooking time
about 15 minutes

200g/7oz broccoli, cut into small florets

575g/1¼lb lean pork steaks, trimmed of visible fat

Fry Light for spraying

1 tsp finely grated fresh root ginger

2 red onions, peeled and sliced

1 yellow pepper, cored, deseeded and roughly chopped

220g/7½oz can water chestnuts, drained and halved

150g/5oz cherry tomatoes

150ml/¼pt chicken stock, made with Bovril

1 tbsp Dijon mustard

6 tbsp snipped chives

2 tbsp soya sauce

salt and freshly ground black pepper

1 Add the broccoli florets to a pan of boiling water and cook for 2–3 minutes, then drain and set aside.

2 Cut the pork into strips. Lightly spray a large, non-stick wok or frying pan with Fry Light and place over a high heat. Add the pork to the pan with the ginger and stir-fry for 3–4 minutes or until it is cooked to your liking. Transfer to a plate.

3 Add the onions and yellow pepper to the wok or frying pan. Stir-fry for 2–3 minutes, then add the broccoli florets, water chestnuts and cherry tomatoes and stir-fry for 1–2 minutes.

4 Return the pork strips to the pan, and add the stock, mustard, chives and soya sauce. Cook gently for 2–3 minutes. Season to taste and serve immediately, on warmed plates.

original

½ **Sin**

green

8 **Sins**

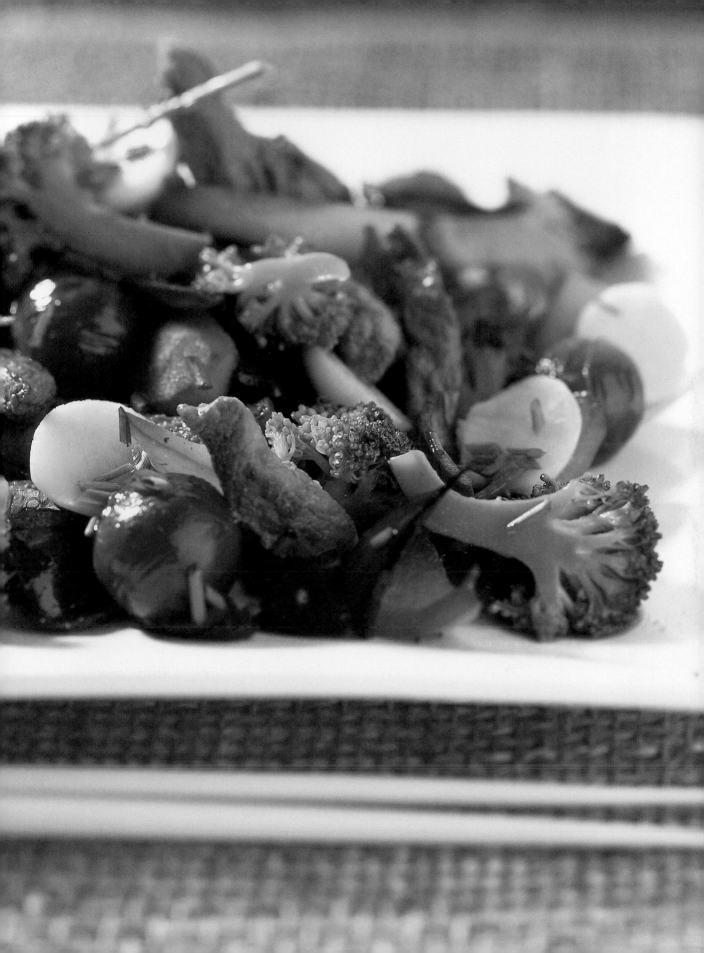

Sweet pepper, pork and pineapple casserole

This simple dish brings together a myriad of contrasting flavours. Seared pork fillet strips, mixed peppers and pineapple chunks are tossed in a tangy, sweet and sour sauce. A mellow parsnip or celeriac mash (see page 114) is the ideal accompaniment.

serves **4**

preparation
10 minutes

cooking time
about 10 minutes

400g/14oz lean pork fillet, trimmed of
    visible fat
1 red pepper
1 yellow pepper
2 tsp sunflower oil
1 garlic clove, peeled and crushed
6 spring onions, sliced diagonally
2 canned pineapple rings, drained and
    roughly chopped
salt and freshly ground black pepper

FOR THE SAUCE:
1 tbsp red wine vinegar
2 tbsp soya sauce
1 tbsp tomato purée
6 tbsp fresh orange juice
1 tsp soft brown sugar
1 tbsp cornflour
TO GARNISH:
snipped chives

1 Cut the pork into thin strips. Halve, core and deseed the peppers, and cut into bite-sized chunks.

2 Mix the ingredients for the sauce together in a bowl until the cornflour is thoroughly blended; set aside.

3 Heat the oil in a large non-stick frying pan. Add the pork to the hot pan and stir-fry for 3–4 minutes or until it is just cooked through. Add the garlic, spring onions and peppers and stir-fry for 2–3 minutes.

4 Add the sauce mixture and pineapple chunks to the pan. Stir and cook for 2–3 minutes until the sauce thickens to coat the pork and vegetables. Season with salt and pepper to taste. Serve immediately, sprinkled with chives.

original

3 Sins

green

8½ Sins

Pork and apple burgers on a wilted spinach salad

Intensely flavoured with parsley, spring onions and thyme, these tasty burgers are kept deliciously moist with the addition of grated apple. Served on a bed of wilted spinach leaves and shredded carrot, they make an inviting lunch or supper dish.

1 large apple

1 bunch of spring onions, trimmed

2 or 3 thyme sprigs

small bunch of flat-leaf parsley, finely
  chopped

675g1½lb lean pork mince

salt and freshly ground black pepper

Fry Light for spraying

FOR THE WILTED SALAD:

100g/3½oz baby leaf spinach

1 large carrot, peeled and shredded

lemon wedges to serve

1 Peel and roughly grate the apple flesh, squeeze out the excess moisture and place in a large bowl. Finely slice the spring onions and mix with the apple. Strip the leaves off the thyme stalks and add them to the mixture with the parsley.

2 Add the minced pork to the apple mixture and mix thoroughly, using your fingers, until well combined. Season with salt and pepper. Divide the mixture into 8 portions and shape into fairly flat burgers.

3 Preheat the grill to medium-hot and line a grill rack with foil. Spray lightly with Fry Light and arrange the burgers on the foil in a single layer. Grill for 5–6 minutes on each side or until cooked through.

4 Meanwhile, heat a large, non-stick wok or frying pan on a high heat and spray with Fry light. When hot, add the spinach leaves and carrot, toss to mix and stir-fry for 1 minute. Season with salt and pepper and remove from the heat.

5 Drain the cooked burgers on kitchen paper. Divide the spinach and carrot mixture between warmed plates. Top each serving with two burgers and serve at once, with lemon wedges.

serves 4

preparation
10 minutes
cooking time
about 12 minutes

original

1 Sin

green

11½ Sins

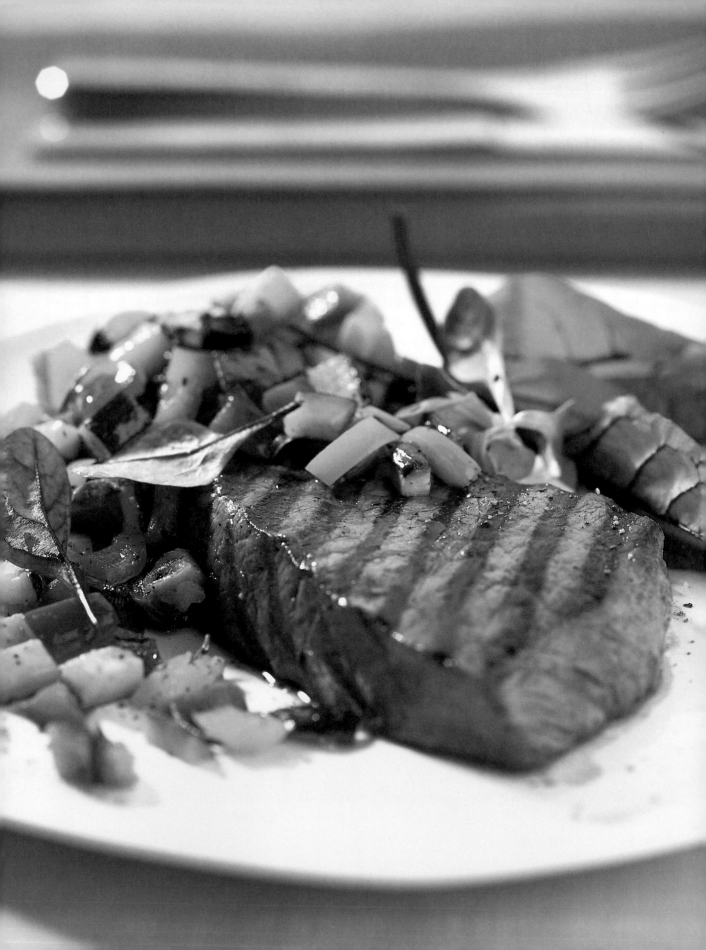

Chargrilled fillet steak with roasted vegetables

Roasted peppers, courgette and aubergine – liberally flavoured with fresh rosemary and garlic – have a mellow sweetness that marries beautifully with juicy, chargrilled fillet steak.

4 lean fillet steaks, each about 175g/6oz, trimmed of visible fat
Fry Light for spraying
1 tsp Worcestershire sauce
salt and freshly ground black pepper
FOR THE VEGETABLES:
1 red pepper, halved, cored and deseeded
1 yellow pepper, halved, cored and deseeded
1 large courgette, trimmed

1 aubergine, trimmed
1 red onion, peeled
1 tbsp olive oil
2 tbsp chopped rosemary leaves
6 garlic cloves, peeled and finely chopped
TO SERVE:
salad leaves
lime or lemon wedges

serves **4**
preparation
10 minutes
cooking time
about 15 minutes

1 First prepare the vegetables. Preheat the oven to 200°C/Gas 6. Cut the peppers, courgette, aubergine and red onion into 1cm/½in dice. Place in a non-stick roasting tin.

2 Sprinkle the oil, rosemary and garlic over the vegetables and toss to mix, then spread out to a single layer and season with salt and pepper. Roast in the hot oven for 12–15 minutes or until just soft.

3 Meanwhile, heat a ridged griddle pan over a high heat. Lightly spray the steaks with Fry Light, then rub with the Worcestershire sauce, season and place on the hot griddle pan. Cook for 2 minutes on each side for medium-rare steaks, or 3–4 minutes each side if you prefer well-done steaks.

4 To serve, place the steaks on warmed plates and spoon on the roasted vegetables. Serve with salad leaves and lime or lemon wedges.

original
1½ Sins

green
13½ Sins

Pan-fried beef with herbs and balsamic vinegar

A powerfully aromatic and rich sauce, flavoured with herbs, balsamic vinegar and garlic, lifts this dish to great heights. Very quick and easy to prepare, it is ideal for a fast, mid-week supper or light lunch. Serve with a fresh tomato and basil salad.

serves **4**

preparation
5 minutes

cooking time
about 15 minutes

4 sirloin steaks, each about 225g/8oz, trimmed of visible fat
1 tbsp chopped rosemary
1 tbsp chopped thyme
1 tbsp chopped oregano
salt and freshly ground black pepper

1 tbsp olive oil
3 garlic cloves, peeled and thinly sliced
175ml/6fl oz balsamic vinegar
400ml/14fl oz chicken stock, made with Bovril

1 Place each steak between two sheets of cling film and beat out to a thickness of about 1cm/½in, using a wooden mallet or rolling pin. Mix the chopped herbs together. Season the steaks and sprinkle with the herbs. Set aside.

2 Heat the olive oil in a large, non-stick frying pan. Add the sliced garlic and cook until it begins to sizzle. Remove with a slotted spoon, drain on kitchen paper and reserve.

3 Place the steaks in the frying pan and cook for 1–2 minutes on each side for medium-rare, or 2–3 minutes for well-done steaks. Transfer them to a warmed plate and keep warm.

4 Pour the vinegar into the pan and bubble rapidly until reduced by half. Add the stock and allow to bubble vigorously for 3–4 minutes or until slightly syrupy.

5 Place the steaks on warmed plates and pour over the sauce. Scatter over the reserved garlic and serve immediately, with a tomato and basil salad.

original
1½ Sins

green
17½ Sins

Creamy beef and mushroom stroganoff

Cocktail gherkins and hot green peppercorns offset the richness of crème fraîche in this stroganoff to bring a new dimension to a traditional favourite. Crisp cooked shredded cabbage makes an excellent accompaniment.

400g/14oz lean fillet steak, trimmed of visible fat

salt and freshly ground black pepper

Fry Light for spraying

1 large red onion, peeled and thinly sliced

250g/9oz button mushrooms, thinly sliced

2 garlic cloves, peeled and crushed

200ml/7fl oz chicken stock made with Bovril

2 tsp green peppercorns in brine, drained

1 tbsp Worcestershire sauce

8 tbsp reduced fat crème fraîche

2 tbsp chopped flat-leaf parsley

60g/2oz cocktail gherkins, drained and chopped

chopped flat-leaf parsley to garnish

serves **4**

preparation

10 minutes

cooking time

about 15 minutes

1 Cut the fillet steak into long, thin strips and season them with salt and pepper. Set aside.

2 Place a large, lidded non-stick frying pan over a medium heat and lightly spray with Fry Light. When hot, add the onion and mushrooms and fry, stirring, for 3–4 minutes.

3 Add the garlic, stock, peppercorns and Worcestershire sauce, cover and simmer for 3–4 minutes. Add the beef strips to the pan, stir and simmer for 3–4 minutes.

4 Stir in the crème fraîche and cook gently for 2–3 minutes. Add the parsley and gherkins and stir to mix. Check the seasoning and serve immediately, garnished with parsley. Accompany with crisp cooked, boiled or steamed cabbage.

Cook's note

To ring the changes, replace the beef with tender strips of lean pork fillet.

original

3 Sins

green

10 Sins

Shish kebabs with kachumber

Lean minced lamb is blended to a paste with yogurt, spices and fresh coriander, then moulded around skewers to make these tasty kebabs. For a special occasion, use lemon grass stalks for skewers – the kebabs will look sensational. A cooling, Indian-style salad is the perfect complement.

serves **4**

preparation

10 minutes

cooking time

8–10 minutes

1.5cm/⅝in cube fresh root ginger, peeled and chopped

1 garlic clove, peeled and chopped

500g/1lb 2oz lean minced lamb

small bunch of coriander

1 tbsp dried mango powder (amchoor), or lemon juice

1 tsp garam masala

1 tsp ground cumin

1 tsp chilli powder

2 tbsp gram (chickpea) flour

2 tbsp very low fat natural yogurt

Fry Light for spraying

FOR THE KACHUMBER:

1 cucumber

4 ripe tomatoes

1 small onion, peeled

1 green pepper, halved, cored and deseeded

juice of 2 limes

1 tbsp chopped coriander leaves

1 tbsp chopped mint leaves

salt and freshly ground black pepper

TO SERVE:

lemon wedges

chopped coriander leaves

1 First make the kachumber. Peel the cucumber, halve lengthways and scoop out the seeds, using a teaspoon. Finely chop the cucumber, tomatoes, onion and green pepper and mix together in a large bowl. Stir in the lime juice and chopped herbs. Season to taste and set aside.

2 To make the kebabs, put the ginger and garlic in a food processor with the lamb. Remove the stalks from the coriander, chop the leaves and add them to the processor with the mango powder or lemon juice. Add the spices, flour and yogurt. Blend to a paste, tip into a bowl and season well with salt and pepper.

3 Preheat the grill. Divide the mixture into 8 portions and mould each into a sausage around a metal skewer. Spray with Fry Light and grill for 8–10 minutes, turning once. Serve immediately, with the kachumber, lemon wedges and a sprinkling of chopped coriander.

original

2 Sins

green

12 Sins

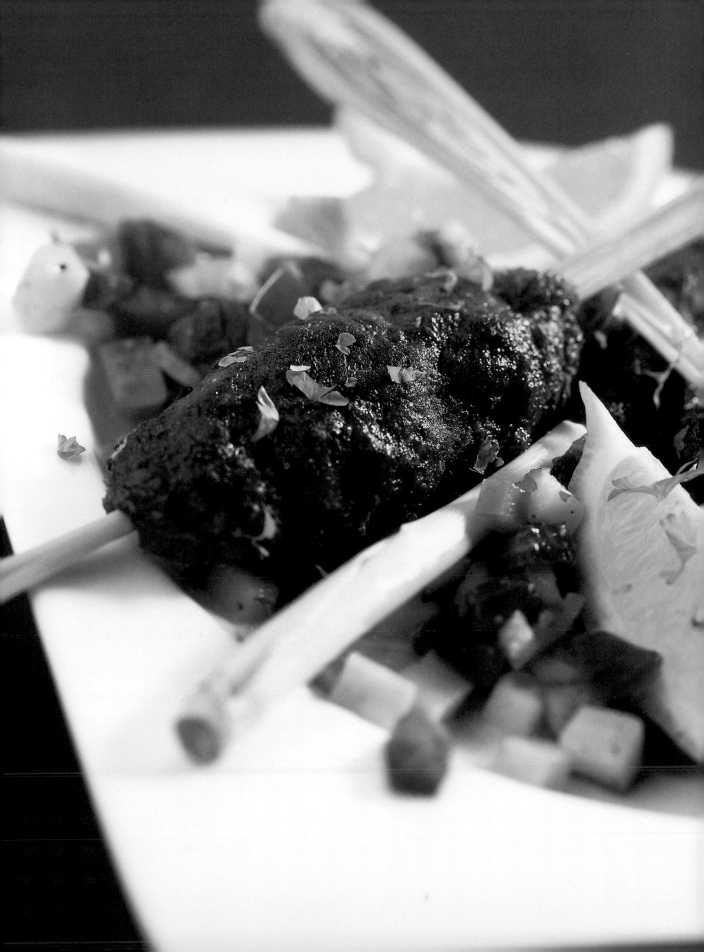

Spicy lamb steaks

Grilled lean lamb steaks are coupled with a spicy tomato, onion and red pepper sauce – bursting with rich flavours and herbs. Served with steamed green beans, this easy dish is great for last-minute entertaining.

serves **4**

preparation

10 minutes

cooking time

about 10 minutes

4 lean lamb steaks, each about 150g/5oz, trimmed of visible fat
Fry Light for spraying
FOR THE SAUCE:
1 onion, peeled and finely chopped
2 garlic cloves, peeled and crushed
2 red peppers, cored, deseeded and finely chopped

1 tbsp chopped oregano
1 tbsp chopped flat-leaf parsley
1 tsp hot paprika
400g/14oz can chopped tomatoes with herbs
1 tsp granulated artificial sweetener
salt and freshly ground black pepper

1   Begin to make the sauce. Place a large, non-stick frying pan on a medium heat and lightly spray with Fry Light. Add the onion and garlic, and stir-fry for 3–4 minutes or until soft. Add the red peppers to the pan with the herbs, paprika, tomatoes, sweetener and seasoning. Bring to the boil and simmer for 5–6 minutes.

2   In the meantime, cook the steaks. Preheat the grill to high. Lightly spray the steaks with Fry Light and place on the grill rack. Cook under the hot grill for 3–4 minutes on each side or until cooked to your liking. Remove and keep warm.

3   Transfer the cooked sauce to a food processor and blend for 1–2 minutes until fairly smooth.

4   To serve, place the steaks on warmed plates and pour the spicy sauce over them. Serve immediately, with steamed green beans.

original

Sin-free

green

10 Sins

Creamy lamb's liver with bacon and onions

The wonderfully warm, mellow flavour and distinctive fragrance of fresh sage transforms this traditional dish of liver and bacon into something special, while the creamy sauce lends a melting richness. Partner with Lime and lemon courgettes (page 162).

serves **4**

preparation
10 minutes

cooking time
12–15 minutes

4 slices lamb's liver, each about 85g/3oz

salt and freshly ground black pepper

Fry Light for spraying

1 large onion, halved, peeled and thinly sliced

6–8 fresh sage leaves, finely shredded

300ml/½pt chicken stock, made with Bovril

4 lean, rindless bacon rashers, roughly chopped

6 tbsp reduced fat crème fraîche

1 Rinse the liver, drain and pat dry with kitchen paper. Season well with salt and pepper and set aside.

2 Place a large, non-stick frying pan over a medium heat and spray with Fry Light. Add the onion and sage, and stir-fry for 4–5 minutes or until soft and lightly browned. Add the stock and bring to the boil, then lower the heat and leave to simmer gently.

3 Place another large, non-stick frying pan on a moderate heat and spray with Fry Light. Add the bacon and stir-fry for 1–2 minutes, then remove with a slotted spoon and reserve. Add the liver to the pan and fry over a moderate heat for 2 minutes on each side or until lightly browned.

4 Add the bacon and liver to the stock mixture and simmer gently for 3–4 minutes or until the liver is cooked but still slightly pink in the centre. Stir in the crème fraîche, taste the sauce and adjust the seasoning. Serve immediately, with lime and lemon courgettes.

original

2½ Sins

green

10½ Sins

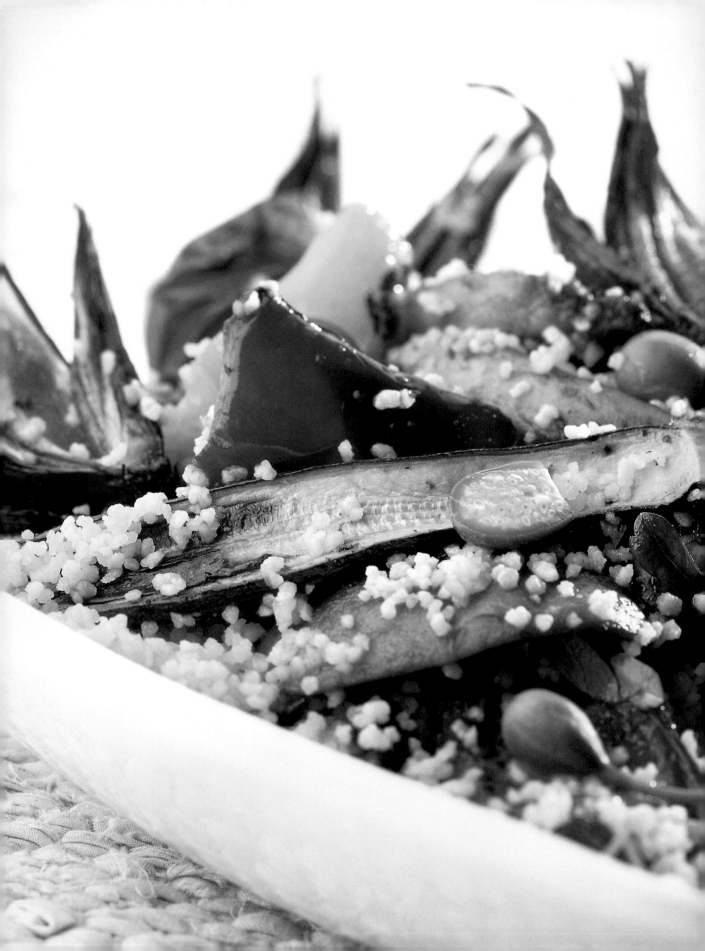

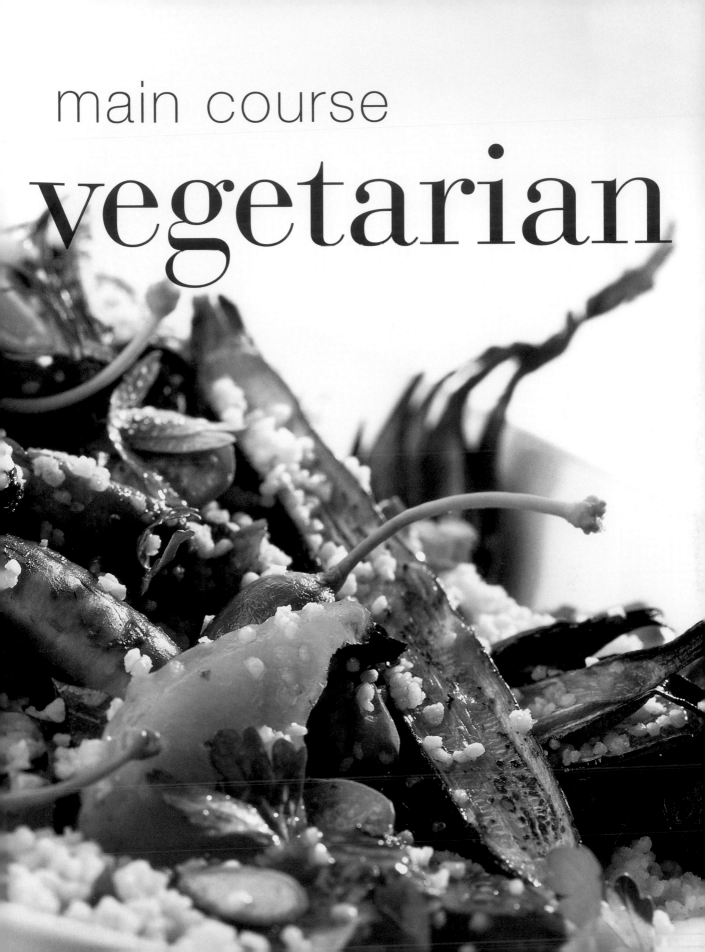

main course
vegetarian

Herb and sweet potato rosti

Rosti are given fresh appeal by using succulent sweet potato, and flavouring the potato cakes generously with parsley and chives. Serve with steamed vegetables or a crisp green salad for a complete meal.

serves **4**

preparation

10 minutes

cooking time

about 20 minutes

✓ vegetarian

500g/1lb 2oz sweet potatoes

300g/10oz potatoes (Desirée or King Edward)

6 spring onions, finely sliced

3 tbsp chopped flat-leaf parsley

3 tbsp chopped chives

1 large egg, lightly beaten

salt and freshly ground black pepper

Fry Light for spraying

1   Peel and coarsely grate the sweet and ordinary potatoes, using a food processor fitted with a coarse grater disc. Transfer to a large sieve and press down with the back of a large spoon to squeeze out as much liquid as possible.

2   Tip the grated potato into a large bowl and add the spring onions, chopped herbs and beaten egg. Season generously, and stir to mix and combine well. Divide the mixture into 4 portions.

3   Place two 15cm/6in non-stick frying pans on a medium heat and spray lightly with Fry Light. When hot, place a portion of the rosti mixture in each pan. Flatten with the back of a spoon to spread evenly and cook for 8–10 minutes on each side, or until cooked through and golden. Using a fish slice or spatula, transfer the rosti to two warmed plates; keep warm.

4   Repeat to cook the remaining two rosti portions. Serve immediately, with steamed green vegetables or a salad.

original

7 Sins

green

Sin-free

Oriental tofu omelettes

Delicious and easy to prepare, these tofu and spring onion omelettes are served with an unusual sauce of rice wine, hoisin sauce, garlic, peas and carrots.

600g/1¼lb silken tofu

3 large eggs, lightly beaten

6 spring onions, finely sliced

salt and freshly ground black pepper

Fry Light for spraying

FOR THE SAUCE:

175ml/6fl oz vegetable stock

2 tbsp hoisin sauce

2 tbsp rice wine or sweet sherry

1 garlic clove, peeled and finely grated

100g/3½oz shelled peas

60g/2oz carrot, peeled and finely diced

serves **4**

preparation

10 minutes

cooking time

about 20 minutes

✓ vegetarian

1 Preheat the oven to low. Place the tofu in a large bowl and mash thoroughly, using a large fork. Add the eggs with the spring onions. Season and mix well.

2 Spray a large, non-stick frying pan with Fry Light and heat until very hot. Cook a quarter of the tofu mixture at a time: spoon half into each side of the pan, to make two small omelettes, keeping them well apart. Cook for 3–4 minutes on each side until golden brown, turning them carefully with a fish slice or spatula, as the mixture is inclined to break up.

3 Transfer the omelettes to a heatproof plate and place in the oven to keep warm. Repeat the process three more times, to make 8 omelettes in total.

4 To make the sauce, add the stock to the frying pan and bring to the boil. Stir in the remaining ingredients, bring back to the boil and simmer for 2–3 minutes until the peas and carrot are tender.

5 To serve, place two omelettes on each plate and pour the sauce over them. Serve at once, with boiled or steamed rice if you like (adding 2 Sins per 30g/1oz on the Original choice).

original

2½ Sins

green

1½ Sins

Cook's note

Fresh silken tofu is sold chilled in most supermarkets and health food shops.

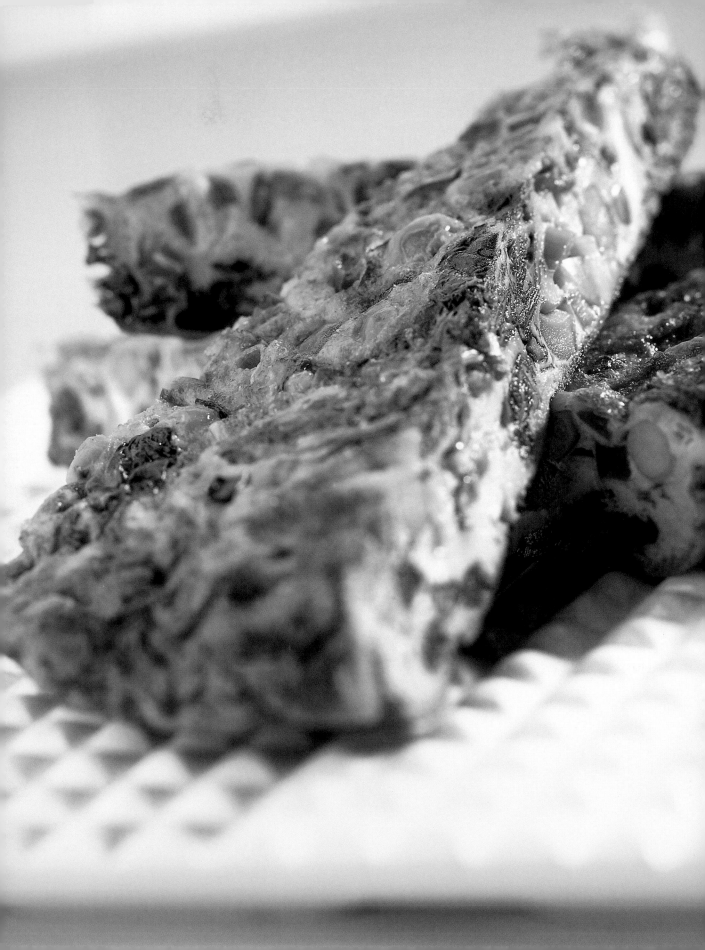

Spinach, pea and mint frittata

Quick and easy to make. this frittata can even be made a day in advance and refrigerated overnight. Bring back to room temperature or heat through before serving. with a crisp green salad.

Fry Light for spraying

4 spring onions, thinly sliced

200g/7oz spinach leaves, washed and
    drained

1 red pepper, cored, deseeded and finely
    chopped

100g/3½oz frozen or fresh shelled peas

3 tbsp chopped mint leaves

6 large eggs, beaten

30g/1oz Parmesan or pecorino cheese, finely
    grated

salt and freshly ground black pepper

serves **4**

preparation

10 minutes, plus

standing

cooking time

15–20 minutes

✓ vegetarian

1 Spray a large, 25cm/10in non-stick frying pan (suitable for use under the grill) with Fry Light and place over a moderate heat. Add the spring onions to the pan and cook gently for 2–3 minutes.

2 Meanwhile, finely chop the spinach. Add to the pan with the red pepper and peas, and cook for 3–4 minutes until the spinach has wilted.

3 Stir the chopped mint into the beaten eggs, then pour into the frying pan. Fry gently for 5–6 minutes or until the base is lightly browned and set.

4 Preheat the grill to medium-hot. Sprinkle the cheese over the surface of the frittata and season with salt and pepper. Place the pan under the grill for 4–5 minutes or until the top is set and golden. Leave to stand for 5 minutes before turning out of the pan. Serve cut into thick wedges, with a crisp green salad.

original

2½ Sins

green

1½ Sins

Bean and mushroom burgers

Hungry children love to tuck into these hearty, lightly spiced vegetarian burgers, made with wholesome ingredients. Serve them with steamed green vegetables and baked potatoes, or a green salad if you prefer.

serves **4**

preparation
10 minutes

cooking time
about 20 minutes

✓ vegetarian

Fry Light for spraying

200g/7oz chestnut or button mushrooms, finely chopped

salt and freshly ground black pepper

400g/14oz can borlotti beans

1 onion, peeled and finely chopped

1 garlic clove, peeled and finely chopped

1 green chilli, deseeded and finely chopped

small bunch of coriander, stalks removed

350g/12oz pack Quorn mince

2 medium eggs, beaten

1 Spray a large, non-stick frying pan with Fry Light. Add the chopped mushrooms, season and stir-fry on a high heat for 4–5 minutes. Take off the heat.

2 Drain the beans thoroughly, place in a large bowl and roughly mash with a potato masher or fork. Add the onion, garlic, chilli and mushrooms.

3 Finely chop the coriander leaves and add them to the bean mixture with the Quorn mince. Add the beaten eggs and stir to mix well. Season and divide the mixture into 8 portions. Shape each portion into a flattish burger.

4 Heat a large, non-stick frying pan and spray the burgers on both sides with Fry Light. When the pan is hot, add the burgers and cook for 6–7 minutes on each side, until lightly browned and crisp. Drain on kitchen paper and serve immediately, with steamed green vegetables and a baked potato, or a salad.

original

8½ Sins

green

Sin-free

Tex Mex chilli

Quorn takes the place of meat in this fast, healthy vegetarian version of a family favourite. Serve it as a sustaining supper, with baked potato wedges or rice, and a crisp green salad.

350g/12oz Quorn pieces

1 red onion, peeled and finely chopped

1 red pepper, cored, deseeded and finely chopped

2 garlic cloves, peeled and finely sliced

2 x 400g/14oz cans red kidney beans, drained

2 x 400g/14oz cans chopped tomatoes

2 tbsp tomato purée

1 tbsp granulated artificial sweetener

2 tsp paprika

2 tbsp chopped flat-leaf parsley

salt and freshly ground black pepper

1 Place the Quorn pieces in a large, non-stick saucepan with the chopped onion, red pepper and garlic. Add the kidney beans, chopped tomatoes, tomato purée, sweetener and paprika and stir to mix.

2 Bring to the boil, stirring occasionally, and cook over a medium heat for about 15 minutes. Stir in the parsley and season with salt and pepper to taste.

3 Serve immediately, or leave to cool and chill overnight so that the flavours have time to develop – reheat the following day to serve. Accompany with baked potato wedges or boiled rice, and a crisp green salad.

Cook's note

To prepare potato wedges to accompany the chilli, preheat oven to 200°C/Gas 6. Cut 2 large baking potatoes into thick wedges, lightly spray with Fry Light, season with sea salt and bake in the hot oven for 20–25 minutes until crisp on the surface and cooked through. (These would be Sin-free on the Green choice.)

serves **4**

preparation
10 minutes

cooking time
15–20 minutes

✓ vegetarian

original

11 Sins

green

½ Sin

Vegetable balti

Balti is always a favourite on the take-away menu, but you can easily make your own delicious, healthy version at home and this recipe is virtually Sin-free on a Green day. Serve with boiled or steamed rice.

serves **4**

preparation

10 minutes, plus

standing

cooking time

about 20 minutes

✓ vegetarian

3 large carrots, peeled

200g/7oz swede, peeled

1 onion, peeled and finely chopped

300g/10oz green beans, trimmed and halved

1 red pepper, cored, deseeded and roughly
    chopped

300ml/½pt vegetable stock

2 garlic cloves, peeled and grated

1 tsp finely grated fresh root ginger

1 tbsp medium curry powder

400g/14oz can chopped tomatoes

2 tsp granulated artificial sweetener

200g/7oz frozen peas

salt and freshly ground black pepper

4 tbsp chopped coriander leaves

TO SERVE:

coriander sprigs to garnish

lemon or lime wedges

very low fat natural yogurt

1 Cut the carrots and swede into bite-sized chunks and place in a large saucepan with the onion, green beans and red pepper. Add the stock, garlic, ginger and curry powder. Bring to the boil and cook over a medium heat for 8–10 minutes, stirring occasionally.

2 Stir in the chopped tomatoes, sweetener and frozen peas, season generously and bring back to the boil. Simmer, uncovered, for 5–6 minutes.

3 Let the balti stand for 5 minutes, then stir in the chopped coriander. Serve immediately, garnished with coriander sprigs. Accompany with very low fat natural yogurt, lemon or lime wedges, and steamed or boiled rice. (Rice counts as 2 Sins per 30g/1oz on the Original choice.)

original

2 Sins

green

negligible

Cook's note
This dish freezes well, so make extra to have as a quick standby meal.

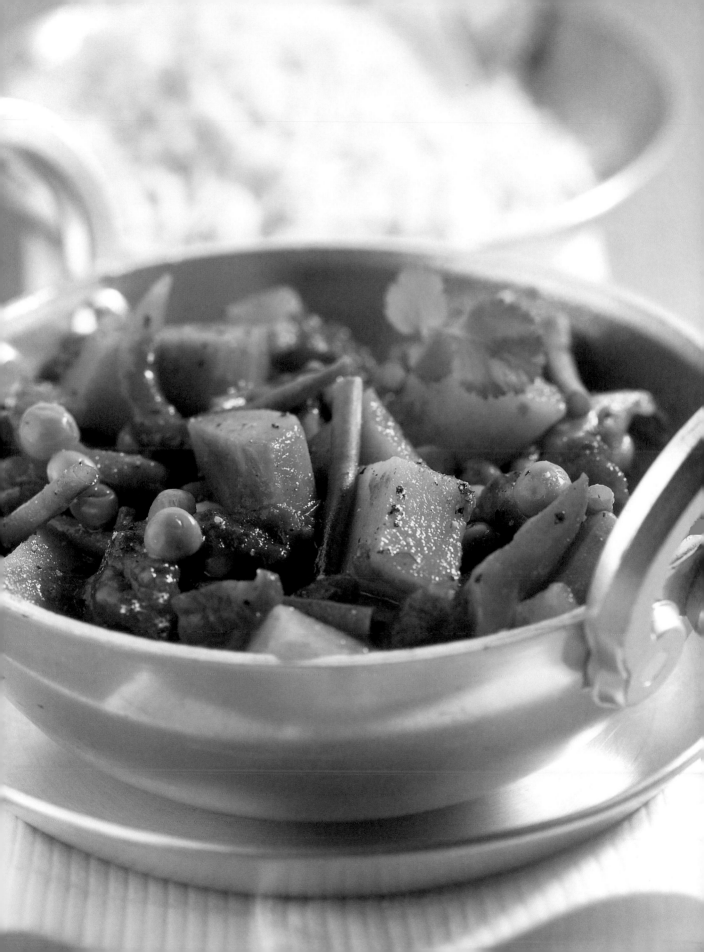

Italian vegetable stew

Root vegetables form the basis for this nourishing stew – ideal comfort food for a chilly winter's evening. If you haven't any fresh oregano, simply substitute flat-leaf parsley.

serves **4–6**

preparation
10 minutes

cooking time
20 minutes

✓ vegetarian

3 small turnips, scrubbed

3 carrots, peeled

250g/9oz parsnips, peeled

400g/14oz new potatoes, scrubbed

1 onion, peeled and finely chopped

3 garlic cloves, peeled and crushed

60g/2oz red lentils

450ml/¾pt boiling-hot vegetable stock

2 x 400g/14oz cans chopped tomatoes

250g/9oz button mushrooms, trimmed

3 tbsp chopped basil leaves

1 tbsp chopped oregano leaves

salt and freshly ground black pepper

1 Roughly chop the turnips, carrots and parsnips. Cut the potatoes into quarters if they are large. Place these vegetables in a large saucepan with the onion, garlic, lentils and hot stock. Stir and bring to the boil.

2 Add the chopped tomatoes and mushrooms and bring back to the boil. Lower the heat and simmer gently for 15 minutes until the lentils are cooked.

3 Remove from the heat and stir in the chopped herbs. Taste and adjust the seasoning. Serve immediately, with rice and a green salad. (Boiled rice counts as 2 Sins per 30g/1oz on the Original choice.)

original

8 Sins

green

½ Sin

Penne arrabiata

For this easy dish, wholemeal pasta is tossed in a thick, rich tomato sauce, spiked with onion, garlic and fresh chilli. You can use regular pasta instead of wholemeal, but you will forfeit the Healthy Extra option on the Original choice.

Fry Light for spraying

1 red onion, peeled and roughly chopped

2 garlic cloves, peeled and finely sliced

1 red chilli, deseeded and finely chopped

400g/14oz passata or creamed tomatoes

3 tbsp chopped basil leaves

1 tbsp chopped oregano leaves

2 tsp granulated artificial sweetener

salt and freshly ground black pepper

350g/12oz dried wholemeal penne

finely grated Parmesan cheese to serve
(optional)

serves **4**

preparation

10 minutes

cooking time

about 20 minutes

✓ vegetarian

1 Lightly spray a large, non-stick frying pan with Fry Light and place on a medium heat. Add the onion, garlic and chilli to the pan and cook, stirring, for 2–3 minutes until softened.

2 Stir in the passata and bring to the boil. Cover the pan and simmer gently for 10 minutes, then add the chopped herbs, sweetener and seasoning, and cook for a further 5–6 minutes.

3 While the sauce is simmering, cook the pasta. Add to a pan of boiling salted water and cook according to the packet instructions until *al dente*. Drain thoroughly.

4 Add the pasta to the arrabiata sauce and toss gently to mix. Serve straight away, in warmed pasta bowls or plates. Sprinkle over some finely grated Parmesan cheese if desired, and accompany with a salad.

Cook's note
For a Sin-free option on the Green choice, omit the sprinkling of Parmesan.

original

15 Sins

green

½ Sin

Linguini with spring greens, garlic and chilli

Not for the faint-hearted, this quick-to-prepare, fiery pasta dish with its powerful aromatic flavours is perfect for a replenishing supper. Wholemeal spaghetti can replace the regular kind to add a Healthy Extra option on an Original day.

serves **4**

preparation
10 minutes

cooking time
about 10 minutes

✓ vegetarian

350g/12oz dried linguine or spaghetti

1 tbsp olive oil

2 large red chillies, deseeded and finely sliced

4–5 garlic cloves, peeled and thinly sliced

200g/7oz spring greens, washed and drained

salt and freshly ground black pepper

30g/1oz pecorino or Parmesan cheese, finely grated

1 Add the linguine to a pan of boiling salted water and cook according to the packet instructions until *al dente*.

2 While the pasta is cooking, heat the olive oil in a large, non-stick frying pan. Add the chillies and garlic, and stir-fry for 2–3 minutes until the garlic turns golden.

3 Finely shred the spring greens and add them to the frying pan. Stir-fry for 5–6 minutes or until the greens have wilted and are just tender.

4 Drain the cooked pasta, add to the frying pan and toss to mix. Season to taste and serve immediately, sprinkled with the grated cheese.

Cook's note
As an alternative to the spring greens, you can use baby leaf spinach, reducing the stir-frying time accordingly. You can also substitute 1 teaspoon dried red chilli flakes for the fresh chilli.

original

18 Sins

green

3 Sins

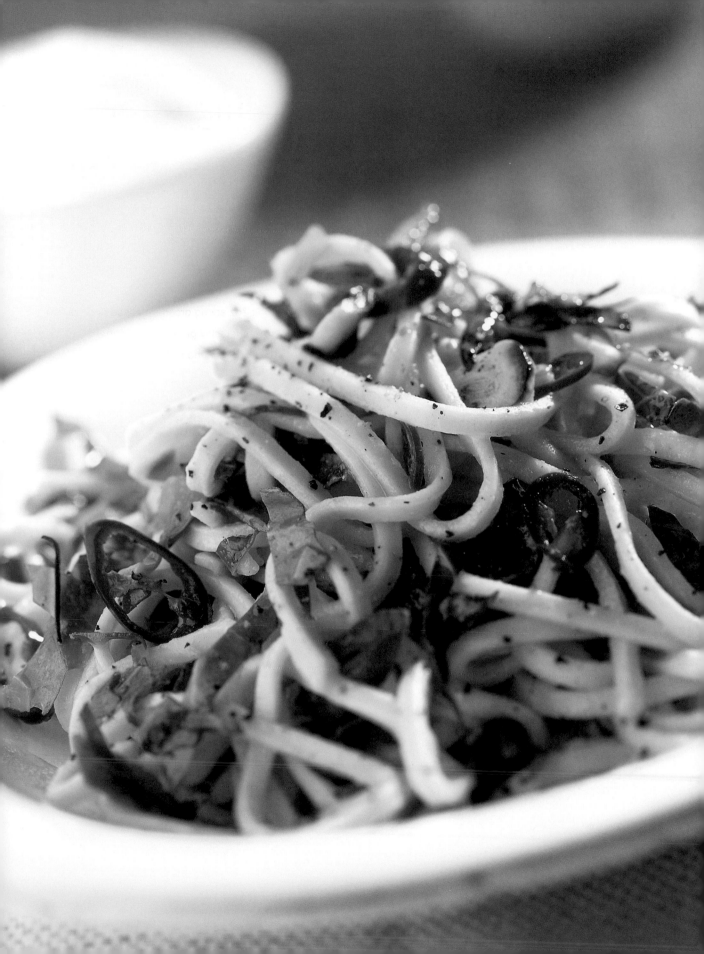

Spaghetti with courgette and cherry tomato sauce

Finely grated courgette – cooked with garlic, tomatoes, fromage frais and basil – makes a delicious, quick creamy sauce for pasta.

serves **4**

preparation
10 minutes

cooking time
about 10 minutes

✓ vegetarian

200g/7oz cherry tomatoes

1 courgette, trimmed

350g/12oz dried spaghetti

1 tbsp olive oil

1 garlic clove, peeled and crushed

1 bunch of basil, stalks removed

2 tbsp very low fat natural fromage frais

6 spring onions, finely sliced

salt and freshly ground black pepper

basil leaves to garnish

1 Finely chop half of the cherry tomatoes; cut the rest in half and reserve. Coarsely grate the courgette, squeeze out the excess liquid, then set aside.

2 Add the spaghetti to a pan of boiling salted water and cook according to the packet instructions until *al dente*.

3 While the pasta is cooking, heat the olive oil in a large, non-stick frying pan. Add the garlic and grated courgette and cook gently for 3–4 minutes, stirring frequently. Add the halved cherry tomatoes and cook for 2–3 minutes.

4 In the meantime, roughly chop the basil and place in a bowl with the fromage frais, spring onions and chopped cherry tomatoes. Stir to mix and add to the frying pan. Season with salt and pepper and toss well.

5 Drain the cooked spaghetti and divide between 4 warmed bowls. Spoon over the courgette and tomato sauce, garnish with basil leaves and serve at once.

original

16½ Sins

green

1½ Sins

Aubergine and pasta gratin

In this simple version of the Italian classic dish, aubergines are cooked with tomatoes, peppers and herbs, tossed with cooked pasta and finished off with a creamy mozzarella topping. Serve with a mixed leaf salad.

300g/10oz dried penne or fusilli

1 red onion, peeled and finely chopped

2 red peppers, cored, deseeded and finely chopped

150ml/¼pt vegetable stock

1 large aubergine, trimmed

2 x 400g/14oz cans chopped tomatoes

3 tbsp chopped basil leaves

salt and freshly ground black pepper

175g/6oz reduced fat mozzarella cheese, grated

1 Add the pasta to a pan of boiling salted water and cook according to the packet instructions until *al dente*. Drain thoroughly.

2 While the pasta is cooking, put the onion and red peppers in a large, non-stick saucepan with the stock. Bring to the boil, cover and simmer for 5 minutes.

3 Meanwhile, cut the aubergine into 3cm/1¼in pieces. Add to the pepper mixture with the tomatoes and chopped basil. Season, bring to the boil and cook over a medium heat for 10 minutes.

4 Preheat the grill to high. Add the cooked pasta to the sauce with half of the mozzarella. Toss to mix and transfer to a shallow ovenproof dish. Sprinkle the remaining cheese over the surface and place under the hot grill for 4–5 minutes until the mozzarella has melted. Serve immediately, with a mixed green salad.

Cook's note

To ring the changes, you could substitute 2 courgettes for the aubergine.

serves **4**

preparation

10 minutes

cooking time

about 20 minutes

✓ vegetarian

original

17 Sins

green

4½ Sins

Pappardelle primavera

Tender green vegetables, tossed in a fragrant herb sauce, are coupled with ribbon pasta to make an effortless mouth-watering supper or lunch. Spaghetti can be used rather than pappardelle or fettuccini if you prefer.

serves **4**

preparation
10 minutes

cooking time
about 10 minutes

✓ vegetarian

350g/12oz dried pappardelle or fettuccini

1 small carrot, peeled and cut into fine matchstick strips

400g/14oz thin asparagus tips

1 courgette, cut into thin batons

100g/3½oz sugar snap peas, trimmed and halved lengthways

2 tbsp reduced fat crème fraîche

2 garlic cloves, peeled and finely grated

4 tbsp chopped fresh mixed herbs (tarragon, flat-leaf parsley and chervil)

salt and freshly ground black pepper

4 spring onions, trimmed and finely shredded

1 Add the pasta to a pan of boiling salted water and cook according to the packet instructions until *al dente*.

2 While the pasta is cooking, add the carrot, asparagus tips, courgette and sugar snaps to a pan of boiling water and cook for 3–4 minutes.

3 In the meantime, mix together the crème fraîche, garlic and chopped herbs. Season with salt and pepper to taste.

4 Drain the vegetables and place in a large bowl with the spring onions. Drain the cooked pasta thoroughly and add to the vegetables with the crème fraîche mixture. Toss to mix and serve immediately.

Cook's note
For a Sin-free meal on a Green day, replace the crème fraîche with very low fat natural fromage frais.

original

16 Sins

green

1 Sin

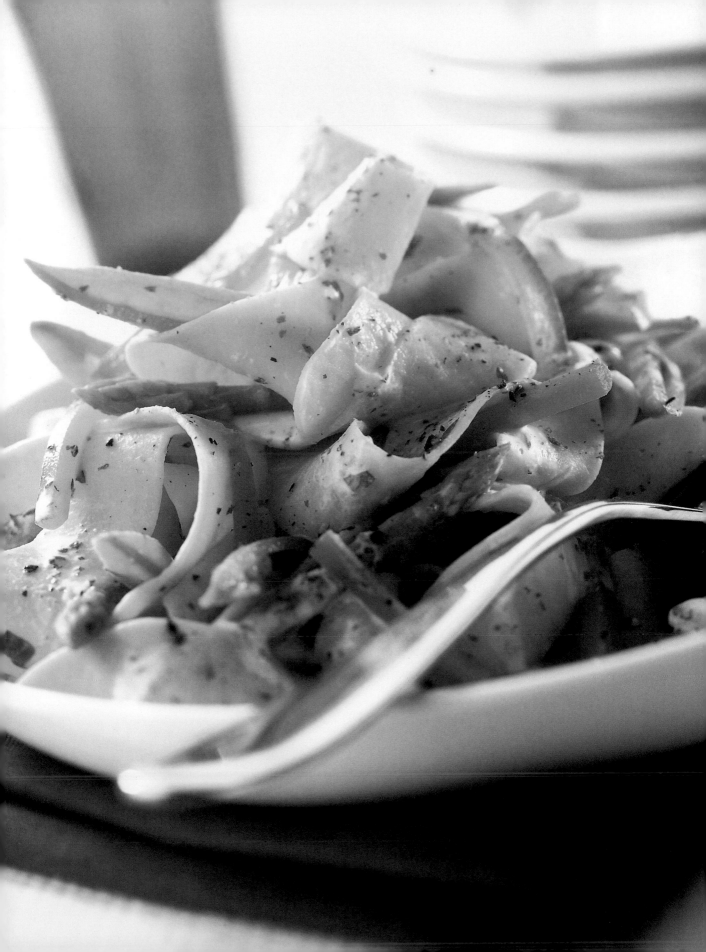

Orange and ginger noodles

Aromatic ginger, soya sauce and orange juice flavour this colourful, sustaining dish of egg noodles, shiitake mushrooms, baby corn and red pepper.

serves **4**

preparation
10 minutes

cooking time
about 7 minutes

✓ vegetarian

6 spring onions, trimmed

100g/3½oz baby corn

340g/12oz dried thick egg noodles

Fry Light for spraying

2.5cm/1in piece fresh root ginger

300g/10oz shiitake mushrooms, thinly sliced

1 red pepper, cored, deseeded and thinly
     sliced

3 tbsp dark soya sauce

juice of 1 orange

4 tbsp chopped chives

salt and freshly ground black pepper

1 Cut the spring onions diagonally into 2.5cm/1in lengths. Halve the baby corn lengthways.

2 Bring a large saucepan of water to the boil and cook the noodles according to the packet instructions.

3 Meanwhile, lightly spray a large, non-stick wok or frying pan with Fry Light and place over a high heat. Add the ginger, spring onions, baby corn, mushrooms and red pepper, and stir-fry for 5 minutes or until the vegetables are tender. Drain the noodles as soon as they are cooked.

4 Add the soya sauce to the vegetables and stir-fry for 1 minute. Add the noodles and orange juice, toss to mix and heat through. Sprinkle over the chopped chives, season to taste and serve immediately, in warmed bowls.

original

17 Sins

green

½ Sin

Vegetable chow mein

Noodles are popular throughout south-east Asia. Here they are tossed with stir-fried spring onions, shiitake mushrooms, carrots, broccoli, mangetout and beansprouts, flavoured with soya sauce and garlic.

serves **4**

preparation
10 minutes

cooking time
about 10 minutes

✓ vegetarian

Fry Light for spraying

2 garlic cloves, peeled and finely chopped

8 spring onions, trimmed and finely chopped

2 tbsp Worcestershire sauce

2 tbsp dark soya sauce

3 large carrots, peeled and cut into thin matchsticks

250g/9oz shiitake mushrooms, finely sliced

250g/9oz broccoli, cut into florets

200g/7oz mangetout, thinly sliced

250g/9oz beansprouts

150g/5oz dried medium egg noodles

salt and freshly ground black pepper

1 Lightly spray a large, non-stick wok or frying pan with Fry Light and place over a medium heat. Add the garlic and spring onions, and stir-fry for 2–3 minutes. Add the Worcestershire and soya sauces, and stir-fry for 2–3 minutes.

2 Add the carrots, mushrooms, broccoli florets and mangetout, together with the beansprouts. Stir-fry over a high heat for 4–5 minutes, or until the vegetables are just tender.

3 Meanwhile, cook the noodles according to the packet instructions. Drain the cooked noodles, add to the vegetables and toss to mix well. Season with salt and pepper to taste, and serve immediately in warmed bowls.

original

7 Sins

green

Sin-free

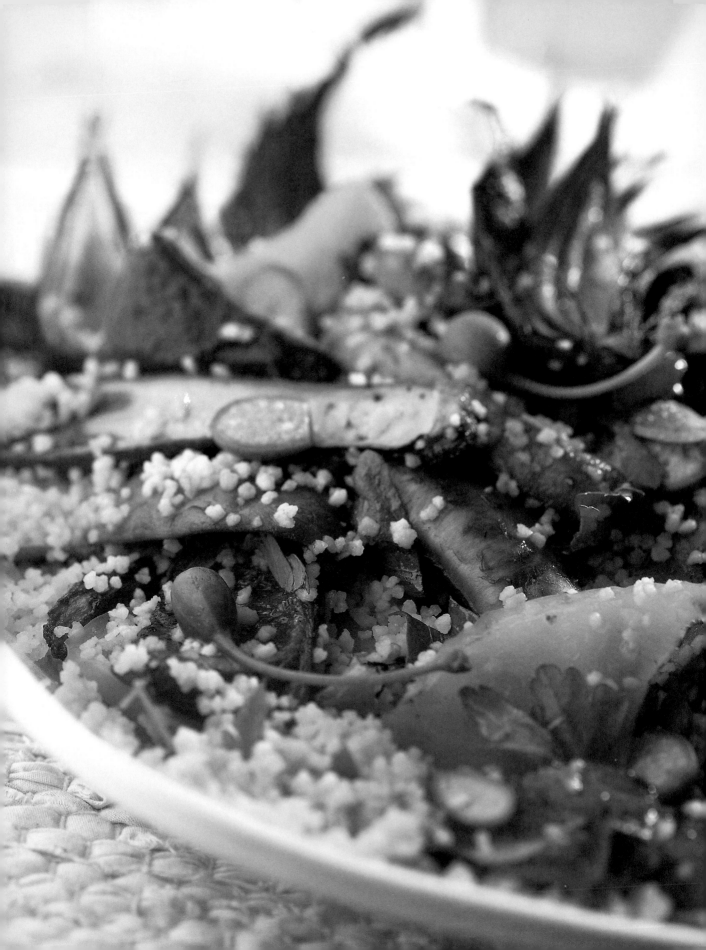

Roasted Mediterranean vegetable couscous

Lightly roasted vegetables, enhanced with herbs and lemon juice, lend a terrific flavour to easy-to-prepare couscous. This inviting supper dish is also good eaten cold and makes a great lunch-box filler the following day... if you have any left over.

Fry Light for spraying

1 large red pepper, halved, cored and deseeded

1 yellow pepper, halved, cored and deseeded

6 baby courgettes, halved lengthways

2 red onions, peeled and quartered

4 large mushrooms, thickly sliced

8–10 medium tomatoes on the vine

3 tbsp chopped rosemary leaves

250g/9oz couscous

450ml/¾pt boiling-hot vegetable stock or water

2 garlic cloves, peeled and finely grated

4 tbsp lemon juice

3 tbsp chopped flat-leaf parsley

100g/3½oz capers or caperberries

salt and freshly ground black pepper

serves **4**

preparation

10 minutes

cooking time

about 15 minutes

✓ vegetarian

1 Preheat the oven to 200°C/Gas 6. Spray a large, non-stick roasting tin with Fry Light. Cut the peppers into bite-sized chunks and place in the roasting tin with the courgettes, onions, mushrooms and tomatoes. Sprinkle with the rosemary and roast in the oven for 15 minutes until just tender.

2 Meanwhile, put the couscous in a large, heatproof bowl and pour over the hot stock or water. Cover the bowl with cling film and leave to stand for 10–12 minutes until all the liquid is absorbed.

3 Mix the garlic and lemon juice together in a bowl. Fluff up the couscous with a fork and toss with the roasted vegetables. Add the garlic and lemon juice mixture, the chopped herbs and capers or caperberries. Season generously, toss lightly and serve immediately.

original

12½ Sins

green

½ Sin

Jewelled tabbouleh

This Middle Eastern dish is delicious served warm, but equally good eaten at room temperature, making it an ideal prepare-ahead entertaining dish.

serves **4**

preparation
10 minutes

cooking time
10–12 minutes

✓ vegetarian

150g/5oz bulghar wheat

4 ripe plum tomatoes

1 red onion, peeled and finely chopped

100g/3½oz canned sweetcorn kernels, drained

1 small bunch of mint

1 small bunch of flat-leaf parsley

juice of 1 lemon

salt and freshly ground black pepper

seeds from 1 pomegranate

lettuce leaves to garnish

1 Put the bulghar wheat in a large saucepan and pour over 1 litre/1¾pts boiling water. Bring to the boil, cover and simmer for 10–12 minutes.

2 Meanwhile, roughly chop the tomatoes and place in a large bowl with the red onion and sweetcorn. Finely chop the herbs and set aside.

3 Drain the bulghar wheat and place in a warmed serving bowl. Fold in the tomato mixture and herbs. Add the lemon juice and season liberally with salt and pepper. Toss gently to mix.

4 Scatter the pomegranate seeds over the tabbouleh and serve warm, garnished with lettuce leaves.

original

7½ Sins

green

Sin-free

Cheesy vegetable and rice to bake

Nutty brown rice and a colourful medley of vegetables – flavoured with tomatoes and fresh herbs – are baked under a cheesy topping to create a rich, warming supper dish. Serve with a refreshing tomato and cucumber salad.

serves **4**

preparation
10 minutes

cooking time
15–20 minutes

✓ vegetarian

1 large courgette, trimmed

150g/5oz green beans, trimmed

150g/5oz broccoli, cut into small florets

150g/5oz cauliflower, cut into small florets

1 large carrot, peeled and thinly sliced

350g/12oz cooked brown rice

salt and freshly ground black pepper

2 tbsp chopped mixed herbs (parsley, thyme and chives)

400g/14oz can chopped tomatoes

115g/4oz reduced fat Cheddar cheese, grated

1 Preheat the oven to 200°C/Gas 6. Bring a large saucepan of water to the boil. Halve the courgette lengthways and slice thickly. Cut the green beans into 3cm/1¼in lengths.

2 Add all of the prepared vegetables to the pan of rapidly boiling water and cook for 3–4 minutes until just tender. Drain.

3 Spread the cooked rice over the base of a medium ovenproof dish and layer the vegetables on top. Season with salt and pepper.

4 Mix the chopped herbs with the tomatoes and spoon over the vegetables to cover them. Sprinkle with the grated cheese and cook in the oven for 10–15 minutes until bubbling. Serve immediately, with a tomato and cucumber salad.

original

10 Sins

green

4 Sins

Chilli and butternut squash risotto

Orange butternut squash, garlic and chilli come together with creamy arborio rice to give you a tempting supper that requires little from the cook, except stirring! A rocket salad is the perfect complement.

serves **4**

preparation and **cooking time**

25–30 minutes

✓ vegetarian

900ml/1½pts vegetable stock

Fry light for spraying

1 red onion, peeled and finely chopped

2 garlic cloves, peeled and finely chopped

1 red chilli, deseeded and finely sliced

250g/9oz arborio or other risotto rice

150g/5oz peeled butternut squash, cut into 1cm/½in dice

salt and freshly ground black pepper

3 tbsp chopped flat-leaf parsley

30g/1oz Parmesan or pecorino cheese, finely grated

1 Bring the stock to the boil in a saucepan over a medium heat. Meanwhile, spray a large non-stick frying pan or saucepan with Fry Light. Add the red onion, garlic and chilli, and cook gently for 2–3 minutes, stirring occasionally.

2 Increase the heat to medium and add the rice to the onion mixture with the chopped butternut squash. Stir in a ladleful of the hot stock.

3 Continue to cook in this manner, adding a ladleful of boiling stock as soon as each addition of liquid is absorbed, stirring constantly. It is essential that the stock is boiling hot as it is added, or the rice will not cook properly. Add the stock in this way until the squash and rice are creamy and *al dente* (tender, but retaining a bite). Season, stir in the parsley and remove from the heat.

4 Ladle into warmed deep plates and sprinkle with grated Parmesan or pecorino cheese. Serve immediately, with a rocket salad on the side.

original

13½ Sins

green

2 Sins

Cook's note
The absorbency of risotto rice varies according to the variety, so you might need to add a little more or less hot stock to obtain the correct consistency.

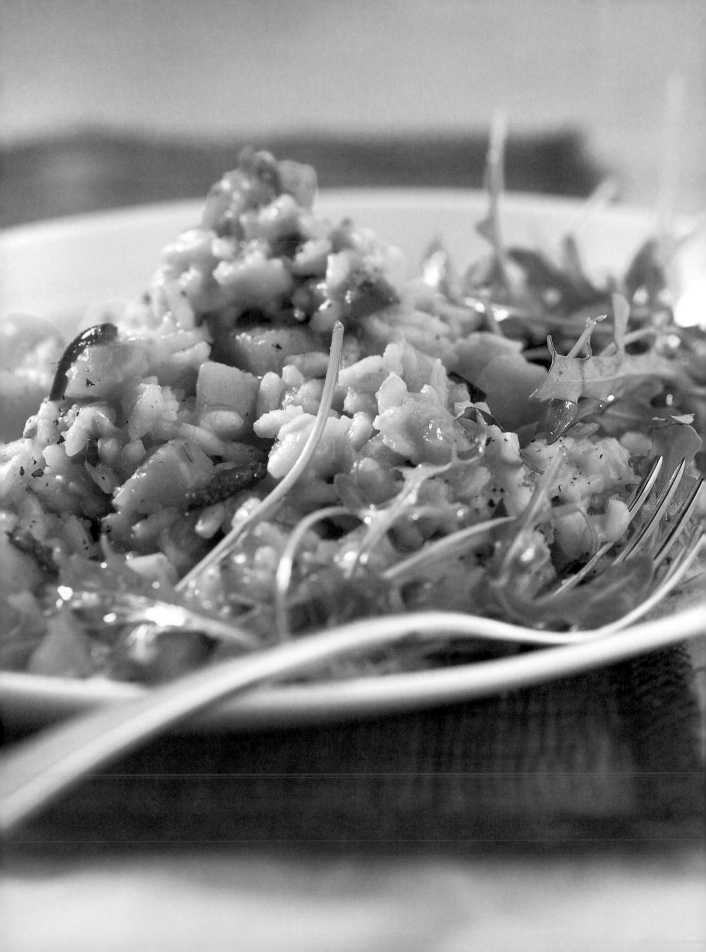

Mixed vegetable pilau rice

Spicy cumin, coriander and red chilli impart a warm glow to this richly flavoured Indian rice dish, while a liberal scattering of fresh-tasting coriander leaves adds fragrance. Brown rice has a nutty flavour and adds fibre, but you can use basmati if you prefer.

serves **4**

preparation and **cooking time**

30 minutes

✓ vegetarian

250g/9oz brown rice

2 large carrots, peeled

200g/7oz broccoli

150g/5oz cauliflower

100g/3½oz peas

Fry Light for spraying

1 large onion, peeled and finely chopped

2 garlic cloves, peeled and crushed

200g/7oz chestnut mushrooms, thinly sliced

1 tsp ground coriander

1 tsp ground cumin

1 red chilli, deseeded and finely sliced

small bunch of coriander, stalks removed

salt and freshly ground black pepper

very low fat natural yogurt to serve

1 Cook the brown rice in boiling water until tender, according to the packet instructions; drain and set aside.

2 Meanwhile, cut the carrots into 1cm/½in dice. Cut the broccoli and cauliflower into small florets. Add to a large pan of boiling water and bring back to the boil. Add the peas and cook for 2–3 minutes or until the vegetables are just tender. Drain and set aside.

3 Spray a large, non-stick wok or frying pan with Fry Light and add the onion, garlic and mushrooms. Stir-fry for 2–3 minutes, then add the ground coriander, cumin and chilli. Stir in the drained vegetables and cook for 2–3 minutes or until heated through. Add the rice and toss to mix well.

4 Finely chop the coriander and add to the pan; season and stir to mix. Serve immediately, with very low fat natural yogurt and a sliced cucumber salad.

original

12 Sins

green

Sin-free

Special vegetable fried rice

The inspiration for this dish comes from the popular Chinese dish. It is always fresh and different, as the vegetables can be varied endlessly, according to what you have in the fridge.

250g/9oz long-grain rice

Fry Light for spraying

2 eggs, beaten

1 red pepper, cored, deseeded and finely chopped

6 spring onions, trimmed and cut into diagonal slices

1 carrot, peeled and cut into matchsticks

100g/3½oz mangetout, thinly sliced

100g/3½oz shelled peas

200g/7oz can sliced water chestnuts, drained

8–10 button mushrooms, sliced

1 garlic clove, peeled and crushed

1 tsp finely grated fresh root ginger

1 tsp mild chilli powder

2 tbsp dark soya sauce

salt and freshly ground black pepper

1 Cook the rice in boiling water according to the packet instructions. Drain, cool and set aside.

2 Meanwhile, spray a large, non-stick frying pan with Fry Light. When hot, pour in the beaten eggs. Lower the heat and cook gently for 8–10 minutes until the base is browned, flip over and cook for a further 3–4 minutes. Remove from the heat and set aside. When cool, cut into thin strips.

3 Put the red pepper, spring onions, carrot, mangetout, peas, water chestnuts and mushrooms in the frying pan. Add the garlic and ginger and stir-fry for 4–5 minutes over a medium-high heat.

4 Add the cooked rice and chilli powder, and stir-fry for 1–2 minutes. Add the egg strips and heat through. Stir in the soya sauce and mix thoroughly. Season with salt and pepper to taste and serve immediately.

Cook's note

This tasty dish is an ideal way to use up leftover cold cooked rice.

serves **4**

preparation
10 minutes, plus cooling

cooking time
about 20 minutes

✓ vegetarian

original

12 Sins

green

Sin-free

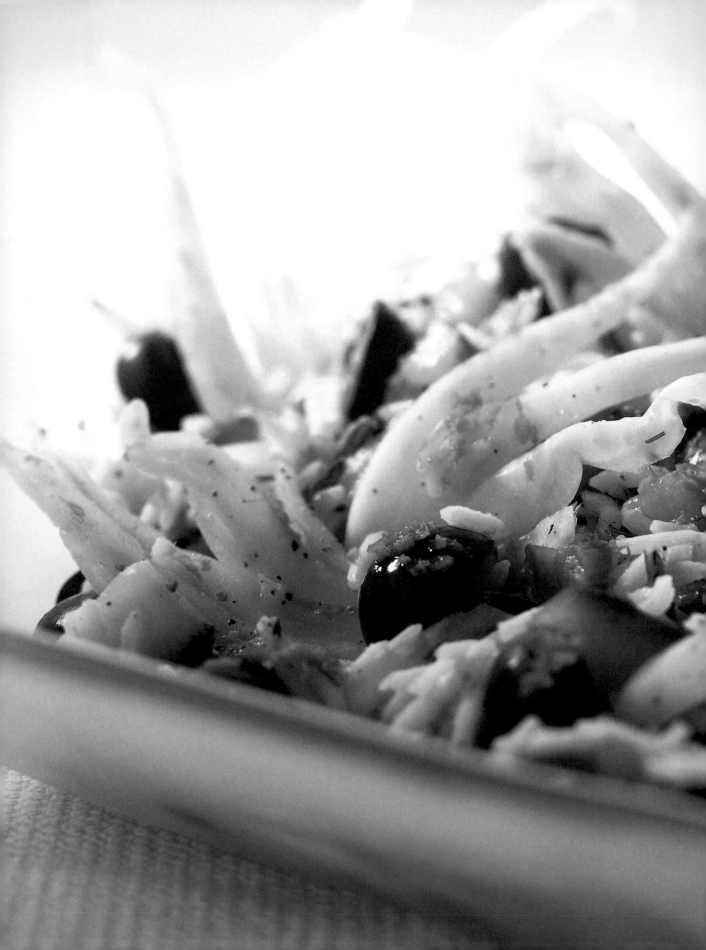

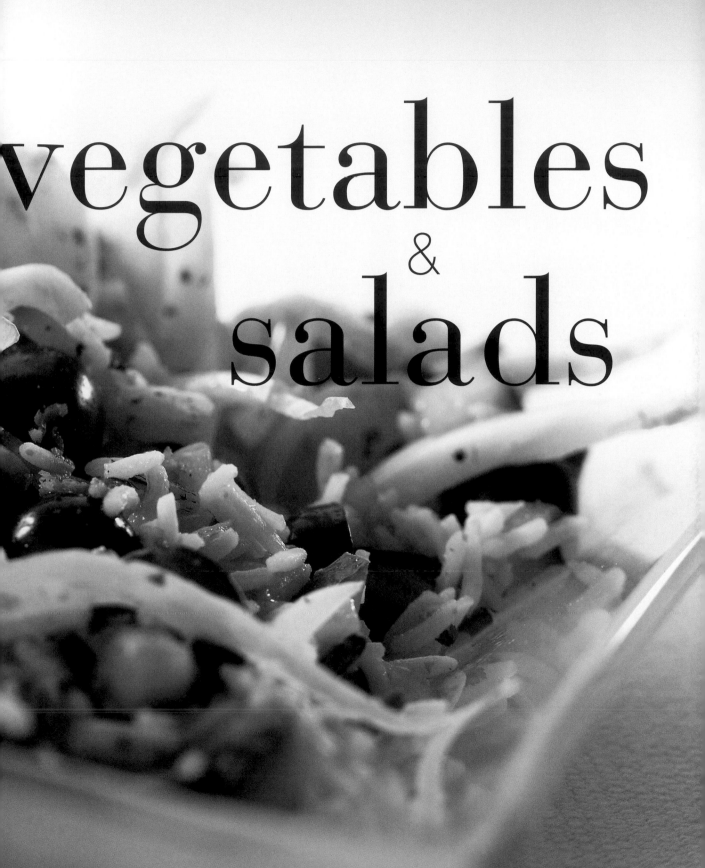

vegetables
&
salads

Stir-fried cabbage with spring greens

Savoy cabbage is suggested for this speedy stir-fry, but you can use curly kale, or white or red cabbage for a different taste and look. Serve with a spoonful of very low fat natural fromage frais, if you like.

serves **4**

preparation

10 minutes

cooking time

6–8 minutes

✓ vegetarian

300g/10oz Savoy cabbage

200g/7oz spring greens

1 tsp olive oil

3–4 garlic cloves, peeled and finely sliced

1 carrot, peeled and coarsely grated

2 tsp caraway seeds

salt and freshly ground black pepper

1 Cut out the core from the cabbage and remove any tough stems from the spring greens. Finely shred the cabbage and greens, keeping them separate.

2 Heat the olive oil in a large, non-stick wok or frying pan. Add the garlic and stir-fry for 30 seconds, then add the Savoy cabbage and stir-fry for 2–3 minutes.

3 Add the carrot and spring greens to the wok and stir-fry for a further 3–4 minutes or until the vegetables are just wilted and the cabbage has turned bright green. The vegetables should be tender but retaining a slight crispness.

4 Sprinkle in the caraway seeds and season generously with salt and pepper. Toss to mix and serve immediately.

original

½ **Sin**

green

½ **Sin**

French-style ratatouille

This roasted ensemble of diced sweet peppers, aubergine, courgettes and cherry tomatoes, scented with garlic and herbs, is a terrific accompaniment to grilled meat or fish. You can also serve it as a light meal in its own right, with salad leaves or a baked potato.

serves **4**

preparation
10–15 minutes

cooking time
15–20 minutes

✓ vegetarian

1 red pepper

1 yellow pepper

2 red onions, peeled

1 small aubergine, trimmed

2 small courgettes, trimmed

Fry Light for spraying

250g/9oz cherry tomatoes

3–4 garlic cloves, peeled and finely chopped

3 tbsp chopped rosemary

3 tbsp chopped basil

salt and freshly ground black pepper

150ml/¼pt vegetable stock

rosemary or basil sprigs to garnish

1   Preheat the oven to 180°C/Gas 4. Halve, core and deseed the peppers, then cut into 1–2cm/½in pieces. Cut the red onions, aubergine and courgettes into 1–2cm/½in cubes.

2   Lightly spray a large, non-stick roasting tin with Fry Light. Place the vegetables in the tin with the cherry tomatoes. Scatter over the garlic and chopped herbs, and season generously with salt and pepper. Pour over the vegetable stock.

3   Cover the roasting tin with foil and bake for 15–20 minutes or until the vegetables are cooked through. Serve garnished with rosemary or basil sprigs.

Cook's notes
● As an alternative to cherry tomatoes, you can use 4–6 quartered plum tomatoes.
● Any leftover ratatouille will make a delicious sauce for pasta.

original

negligible

green

negligible

Lime and lemon courgettes

Tender courgette ribbons – flavoured with tangy citrus zest and fresh mint – make a wonderfully refreshing, simple accompaniment to serve with pan-fried or grilled fish and meat.

serves **4**

preparation

10 minutes

cooking time

3–4 minutes

✓ vegetarian

500g/1lb 2oz courgettes, trimmed

small bunch of mint, stems removed

1 lime

1 small lemon

1 tbsp olive oil

coarse sea salt and freshly ground black pepper

1 Using a vegetable peeler, pare along the length of the courgettes to cut them into long, thin strips. Finely chop the mint leaves and set aside.

2 Finely grate the zest of the lime and half of the lemon. Using the vegetable peeler, pare the zest from the other half of the lemon, cut into julienne strips and set aside for the garnish.

3 Heat the olive oil in a large, non-stick frying pan. When hot, add the courgettes and fry gently, stirring, for 3–4 minutes or until lightly browned and just cooked.

4 Sprinkle the chopped mint and grated citrus zests over the courgettes and toss gently to mix. Season generously with salt and pepper. Serve immediately, sprinkled with the lemon zest julienne.

Cook's note

As you are using the zest, buy unwaxed lemons and limes and wash them thoroughly before grating. Make sure you only grate the coloured outer zest; the white pith would lend an unwelcome bitterness.

original

1½ Sins

green

1½ Sins

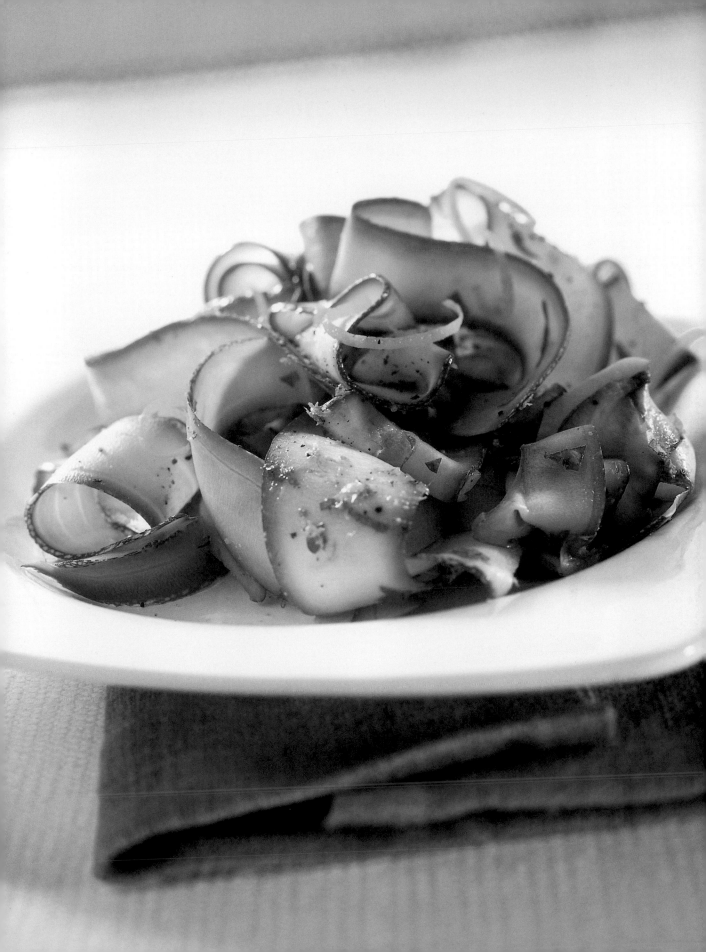

Mixed mushrooms with garlic, lemon and parsley

This harmonious mix of mushrooms, garlic, lemon and flat-leaf parsley makes a great accompaniment to chicken or fish. It can also be served with pasta, as a light lunch dish.

serves **4**

preparation

10 minutes

cooking time

7–10 minutes

✓ vegetarian

500g/1lb 2oz mixed mushrooms (flat, button, chestnut, ceps, chanterelles)

Fry Light for spraying

4 garlic cloves, peeled and finely chopped

salt and freshly ground black pepper

finely grated zest of 1 small lemon

4 tbsp chopped flat-leaf parsley

1 tbsp chopped tarragon (optional)

1 Trim the mushrooms and wipe them clean with damp kitchen paper. Cut the larger mushrooms into thick slices.

2 Spray a large, non-stick frying pan with Fry Light and place on a medium heat. Add the garlic and stir-fry for 1 minute.

3 Add the mushrooms to the pan, season well and cook over a high heat, stirring frequently, for 6–8 minutes or until the mushrooms are lightly browned.

4 Remove from the heat and stir in the grated lemon zest and chopped herbs. Stir to mix, check the seasoning and serve immediately.

Cook's notes
- This is an excellent way to cook wild mushrooms when they are in season.
- To vary the taste, replace the lemon zest with finely grated orange zest.

original

Sin-free

green

Sin-free

Baked stuffed herbed tomatoes

An excellent accompaniment to any meat, chicken or fish dish, these tasty tomatoes are also good served as a light lunch, with a handful of salad leaves. They can be eaten cold, too – the perfect picnic lunch filler.

4 large ripe tomatoes

150g/5oz very low fat natural fromage frais

6 spring onions, finely chopped

2 garlic cloves, peeled and crushed

½ red pepper, deseeded and finely chopped

4 tbsp chopped flat-leaf parsley

salt and freshly ground black pepper

Fry Light for spraying

1 Preheat the oven to 200°C/Gas 6. Cut the tomatoes in half horizontally, then scoop out and discard the seeds. Set aside.

2 Place the fromage frais in a bowl with the spring onions, garlic and red pepper. Add the chopped parsley and mix well, seasoning with salt and pepper to taste. Spoon this filling into the scooped-out tomatoes.

3 Lightly spray a non-stick baking sheet with Fry Light and place the stuffed tomatoes on it. Bake in the hot oven for 10 minutes or until just softened. Serve immediately, or cool, chill and eat the next day.

serves **4**

preparation

10 minutes

cooking time

10 minutes

✓ vegetarian

original

Sin-free

green

Sin-free

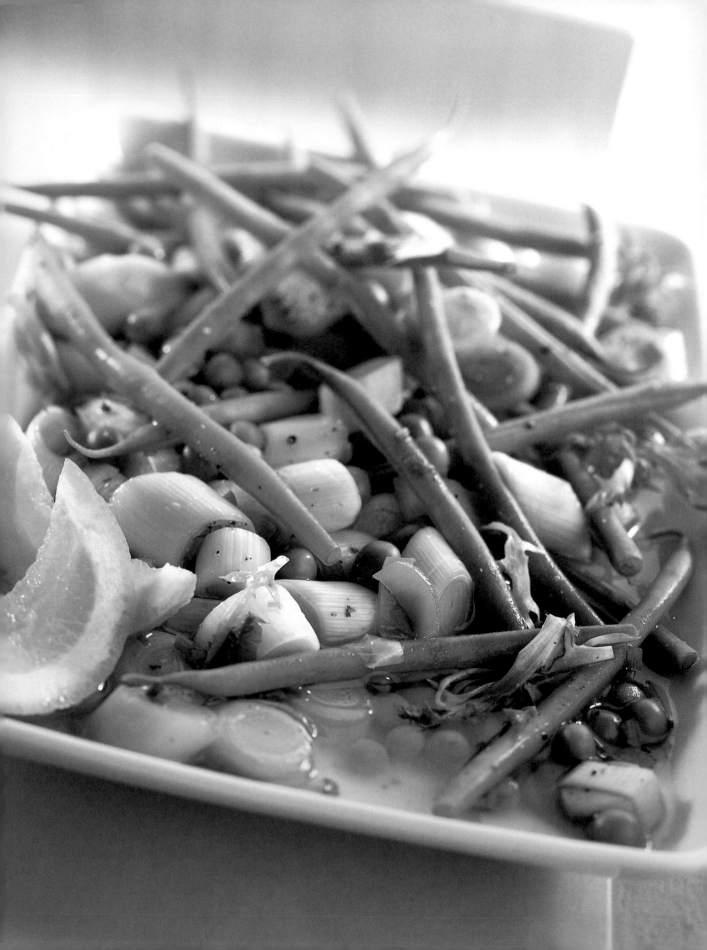

Spring vegetable sauté with herbs

This fresh-tasting sauté of peas, beans and frisée (curly endive) – delicately flavoured with fresh herbs and lemon – makes a delightful accompaniment to grilled and pan-fried fish, chicken and meat.

1 tbsp olive oil

1 garlic clove, peeled and crushed

300g/10oz baby leeks, trimmed and sliced

200g/7oz green beans, trimmed

150g/5oz shelled fresh peas

150ml/¼pt vegetable stock

200g/7oz frisée (curly endive)

1 tbsp chopped mint leaves

1 tbsp chopped chives

1 tbsp chopped chervil

juice of ½ lemon

salt and freshly ground black pepper

lemon wedges, to serve

serves **4**

preparation

10 minutes

cooking time

about 15 minutes

✓ vegetarian

1 Heat the oil in a large, non-stick frying pan. Add the garlic and leeks, and sauté for 3–4 minutes or until the leeks have softened.

2 Add the green beans and peas to the frying pan and continue to sauté for a further 2 minutes.

3 Pour in the vegetable stock, cover and simmer for 5 minutes. In the meantime, separate the frisée leaves and add them to the pan. Continue to simmer for 4–5 minutes. Stir in the herbs and lemon juice, and season with salt and pepper to taste. Serve immediately, with lemon wedges.

original

3 Sins

green

1½ Sins

Cajun-style vegetables

Sin-free whether you are on an Original or Green day, these spiced Creole-style vegetables will complement any simple meat, fish or vegetarian dish.

serves **4**

preparation
10 minutes

cooking time
10–12 minutes

✓ vegetarian

Fry Light for spraying

2 large courgettes, trimmed

1 red pepper, halved, cored and deseeded

1 red onion, peeled

2 plum tomatoes, halved

1 tsp ground Cajun spice seasoning

salt and freshly ground black pepper

FOR THE DRESSING:

1 ripe plum tomato, finely chopped

1 red chilli, deseeded and finely chopped

2 tbsp very low fat natural fromage frais

juice of 1 lime

2 tbsp chopped coriander leaves

1   Preheat the grill to high. Lightly spray a grill pan with Fry Light. Cut the courgettes and red pepper into bite-sized chunks. Cut the red onion into 8 wedges.

2   Arrange the vegetables and tomato halves on the grill pan, and sprinkle with the Cajun spice seasoning. Season generously with salt and pepper. Cook under the preheated grill for 10–12 minutes, turning occasionally.

3   Meanwhile, make the dressing. Mix the ingredients together in a small bowl and season with salt and pepper to taste.

4   Place the grilled vegetables in a warmed large, shallow bowl and pour over the dressing. Toss to mix and serve immediately.

original

Sin-free

green

Sin-free

Creamy dal

In Indian cookery, a variety of lentils, dried beans and split peas are simmered with spices to make dal. In this version, quick-cooking red lentils are infused with spices and aromatics, to make a creamy dal that is delicious served with rice, vegetables and spicy meat dishes.

350g/12oz split red lentils

1.2 litres/2pts boiling water

1 tsp ground turmeric

1 tsp chilli powder

1cm/½in piece fresh root ginger, peeled and finely grated

4 garlic cloves, peeled and finely grated

200g/7oz can chopped tomatoes

1 tsp garam masala

salt

Fry Light for spraying

1 small onion, peeled and finely chopped

1 tsp ground cumin

100g/3½oz cooked mixed vegetables (carrots, green beans and cauliflower), roughly chopped

4 tbsp chopped coriander leaves

serves **4**

preparation

10 minutes

cooking time

about 20 minutes

✓ vegetarian

1   Wash the lentils in a large sieve under cold running water, then place them in a saucepan and pour on the boiling water. Add the turmeric and chilli powder, cover and bring to the boil.

2   Add the ginger and garlic to the saucepan with the chopped tomatoes, and bring back to the boil. Reduce the heat and simmer for 10–12 minutes until the lentils are almost soft and most of the liquid has been absorbed.

3   Stir in the garam masala and season with salt. Simmer, uncovered, for a further 5 minutes.

4   In the meantime, spray a non-stick frying pan with Fry Light and place on a low heat. Add the onion with the cumin, and cook gently, stirring frequently, for 5–6 minutes or until soft.

5   When the dal is ready, add the chopped mixed vegetables, together with the onion. Stir in the coriander, check the seasoning and serve at once.

original

12 Sins

green

Sin-free

Spiced roasted baby new potatoes

Tiny, tender new potatoes – delicately scented with garlic and flavoured with whole, crushed spices – are roasted to golden perfection. This simple accompaniment can be prepared in next to no time.

serves **4**

preparation

5 minutes

cooking time

20–25 minutes

✓ vegetarian

1.5kg/3¼lb baby new potatoes

6 garlic cloves, peeled and thinly sliced

Fry Light for spraying

2 tbsp coriander seeds

2 tbsp cumin seeds

2 tsp onion seeds

1 tsp dried red chilli flakes

coarse sea salt

chopped coriander leaves to garnish

1 Preheat the oven to 200°C/Gas 6. Wash the potatoes, scrub and pat dry on kitchen paper. Line a large baking sheet with baking parchment and place the potatoes on it, in a single layer.

2 Scatter the garlic slices evenly over the potatoes, then lightly spray them with Fry Light.

3 Lightly crush the coriander and cumin seeds using a pestle and mortar, then mix in the onion seeds and dried chilli flakes. Sprinkle this mixture over the potatoes and season with the sea salt. Bake in the hot oven for 20–25 minutes until tender and golden.

4 Transfer to a warmed, large serving bowl and sprinkle with chopped coriander leaves. Serve immediately.

Cook's note
Tiny new potatoes are ideal for this dish. If you can only find larger ones, cut them in half before roasting.

original

13 Sins

green

Sin-free

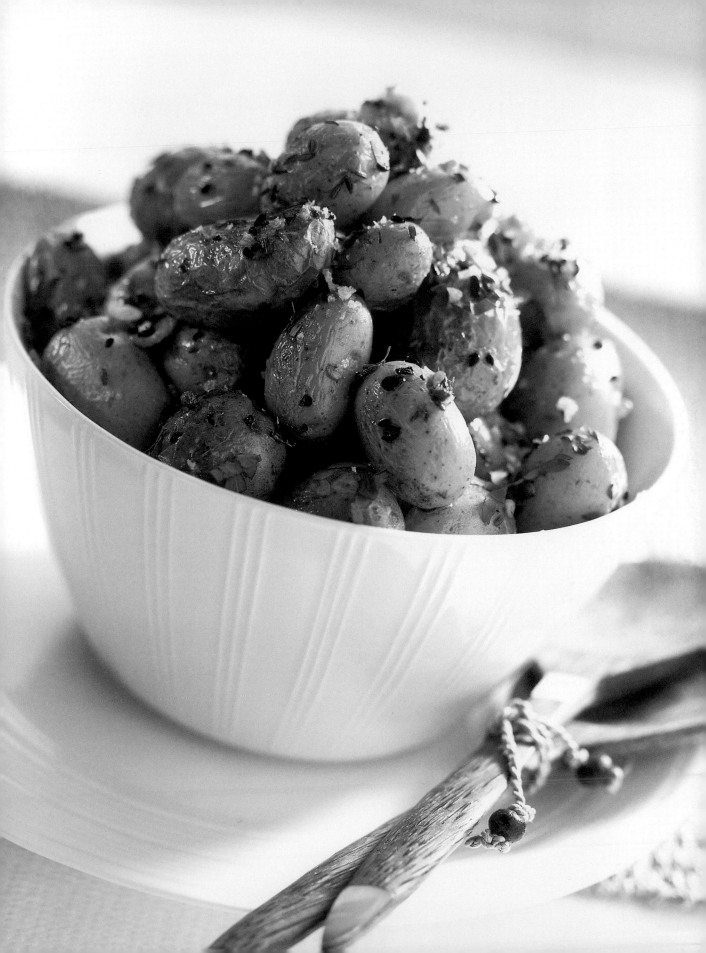

Boulangère potatoes

Baked potato dishes are always popular, and easy to assemble. Here, the potatoes are par-boiled to shorten the baking time, and vegetable stock is used to moisten the bake, rather than cream.

serves **4**

preparation

10 minutes, plus standing

cooking time

20 minutes

✓ vegetarian

750g/1lb 10oz floury potatoes, peeled
225g/8oz onions, peeled and thinly sliced
salt and freshly ground black pepper
freshly grated nutmeg

3–4 garlic cloves, peeled and crushed
350ml/12fl oz boiling-hot vegetable stock
Fry light for spraying

1 Preheat the oven to 220°C/Gas 7. Halve or quarter the potatoes, depending on size, and par-boil for 5–7 minutes. Drain well and slice when they are cool enough to handle.

2 Layer the potato and onion slices in a shallow, ovenproof dish, seasoning the layers with salt, pepper and grated nutmeg to taste. Finish with a liberal sprinkling of seasoning.

3 Stir the garlic into the stock and pour over the potatoes. Lightly spray the surface with Fry light and bake for 20 minutes, or until the top is browned and the potatoes are cooked through. Leave to stand for 5 minutes before serving.

Cook's note
This is a good way to use up leftover cooked potatoes, provided they are not too soft. You can roughly dice the potatoes rather than slice them if you prefer.

original

6½ Sins

green

negligible

Roasted asparagus with a balsamic dressing

Roasting asparagus brings out its full, delectable flavour, and it's a far healthier alternative to boiling and drenching the vegetable in butter. Here, roasted asparagus is drizzled with a rich, garlicky balsamic vinegar dressing – enhanced with caramelised shallots and thyme. Serve warm, or at room temperature if you prefer.

500g/1lb 2oz asparagus, trimmed

Fry Light for spraying

6 large garlic cloves, peeled and quartered

4 shallots, peeled and quartered

5 tbsp water

3 tbsp balsamic vinegar

salt and freshly ground black pepper

2 tbsp chopped fresh thyme

1 Preheat the oven to 220°C/Gas 7. Place the asparagus in a large, shallow ovenproof dish and lightly spray with Fry Light to coat evenly. Roast for 15–20 minutes, depending on the thickness of the spears, until they are softened and lightly browned.

2 Meanwhile, lightly spray a large frying pan with Fry Light and place on a medium heat. Add the garlic and shallots, and stir-fry for 6–7 minutes until golden brown.

3 Add the 5 tbsp water, cover and simmer for 4–5 minutes until softened. Sprinkle with the balsamic vinegar and bring to the boil.

4 Pour the dressing over the hot asparagus, season with salt and pepper to taste, and sprinkle with the chopped thyme. Serve straight away, or set aside for a few hours to allow the flavours to develop, then serve at room temperature.

serves **4**

preparation
10 minutes

cooking time
15–20 minutes

✓ vegetarian

original

Sin-free

green

Sin-free

Fennel and wild rice salad

Grapes and orange add a touch of sweetness to a tempting salad that combines the earthy flavours of fennel and wild rice, with cucumber and spring onion.

serves **4**

preparation
10 minutes

cooking time
15–18 minutes

✓ vegetarian

175g/6oz American easy-cook mixed wild
   rice and long-grain white rice
425ml/¾pt boiling water
salt
1 large cucumber
1 large fennel bulb, trimmed
6 spring onions, trimmed
200g/7oz red or black seedless grapes,
   halved
finely grated zest of 1 orange

FOR THE DRESSING:
juice of 2 oranges
4–5 chervil sprigs
2 tarragon sprigs
1 flat-leaf parsley sprig
2 tbsp red wine vinegar
salt and freshly ground black pepper

1 Place the rice in a medium saucepan and pour over the boiling water. Add salt, bring to the boil, cover and simmer for 15–18 minutes or until the rice is cooked and the water is absorbed.

2 Meanwhile, finely dice the cucumber and cut the fennel and spring onions into very thin slices. Combine these salad vegetables in a bowl. Add the grapes and orange zest, and toss to mix.

3 To make the dressing, pour the freshly squeezed orange juice into a bowl. Finely chop the herbs and add them to the orange juice with the vinegar. Whisk to combine and season with salt and pepper.

4 As soon as the rice is cooked, rinse it briefly under cold water and drain thoroughly. Add to the salad ingredients and mix gently. Pour the dressing over the salad and serve.

original

8 Sins

green

½ Sin

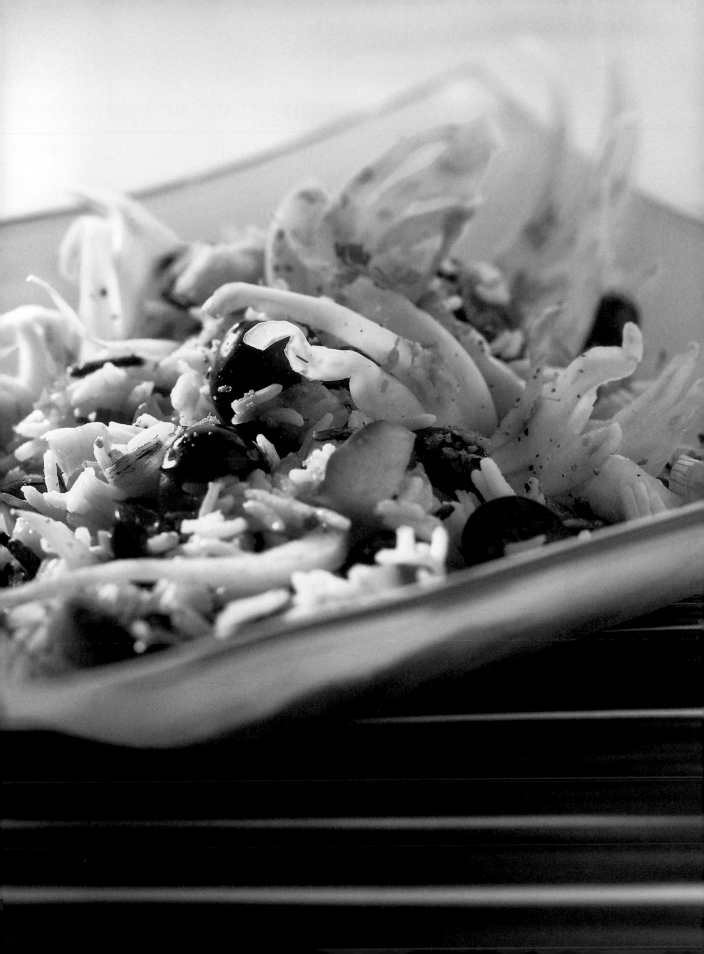

Apple and baby spinach salad

A mustardy, herb dressing and grilled garlic croûtons make great partners for crisp baby spinach leaves and sweet crunchy apples. For a lighter salad, omit the croûtons.

serves **4**

preparation

10 minutes

cooking time

about 6 minutes

✓ vegetarian

2 garlic cloves

2 slices Nimble wholemeal bread, crusts
    removed

2 crisp, red-skinned apples

100g/3½oz baby spinach leaves

FOR THE DRESSING:

6 tbsp chopped mixed herbs (mint, flat-leaf
    parsley and chives)

90ml/3fl oz organic apple juice

2 tsp mild mustard

2 tbsp cider vinegar

salt and freshly ground black pepper

TO GARNISH:

snipped chives or flat-leaf parsley

1   Preheat the grill to high. Place the garlic cloves under the hot grill for 3–4 minutes until the skins are blackened, turning once. Leave until cool enough to handle.

2   Meanwhile, make the dressing. Put all the ingredients in a food processor and blend until smooth.

3   Squeeze out the flesh from the garlic skins into a bowl and mash with a fork. Spread one side of each bread slice with the garlic paste, then cut the slices into 2.5–3cm/1in pieces. Arrange them in a single layer on a grill pan and toast under the hot grill for 1–2 minutes until lightly browned, turning once.

4   In the meantime, quarter, core and slice the apples. Place in a salad bowl with the spinach and toss together. Scatter over the croûtons. Drizzle the dressing over the salad and toss to mix. Serve straight away, garnished with chives or parsley.

original

1½ Sins

green

1½ Sins

Piquant crab salad

An irresistible combination of fresh white crabmeat, creamy cottage cheese, fragrant coriander and crisp vegetables – presented with a spicy dressing and vegetables for dipping. Serve this salad as an elegant lunch or light supper.

¼ cucumber

1 small red onion, peeled and halved

4 spring onions, trimmed

1 fresh red chilli, deseeded

1 small red pepper, halved, cored and
    deseeded

500g/1lb 2oz fresh white crabmeat

100g/3½oz very low fat natural cottage
    cheese

2 tbsp chopped coriander leaves

salt and freshly ground black pepper

FOR THE DRESSING:

3 tbsp reduced fat mayonnaise

6 tbsp very low fat natural fromage frais

1 tsp dried red chilli flakes

TO SERVE:

Little Gem lettuce leaves

celery and carrot sticks

serves **4**

preparation
10 minutes

1 Peel the cucumber, halve lengthways and deseed, then chop finely. Thinly slice the red onion and spring onions. Finely chop the chilli and red pepper. Place all these ingredients in a mixing bowl.

2 Pick over the fresh crabmeat to make sure there are no bits of shell, then add to the salad with the cottage cheese and chopped coriander. Gently mix until evenly combined. Season with salt and pepper to taste.

3 For the dressing, in a small bowl, mix together the mayonnaise and fromage frais, then stir in the chilli flakes.

4 To serve, divide the crab mixture between individual plates. Serve the chilli and mayonnaise dressing on the side, for people to help themselves. Accompany with little crisp lettuce leaves, celery and carrot sticks, to scoop into the crab salad.

Cook's note
If fresh crab isn't available, you could use frozen (and thawed) or canned crabmeat, well drained, instead.

original

2 Sins

green

11 Sins

Prawn and mango salad

Stripy pink prawns are partnered with sweet, juicy mango and bitter salad leaves in a creamy shallot and cider vinegar dressing. This ultra-quick, pretty summer salad is satisfying, but not too rich.

serves **4**

preparation

15 minutes

2 medium, ripe mangoes

100g/3½oz mixed salad leaves (radicchio, frisée, rocket)

400g/14oz cooked, peeled tiger prawns

FOR THE DRESSING:

1 small shallot, peeled

150g/5oz very low fat natural fromage frais

1 tbsp cider vinegar

salt and freshly ground black pepper

TO GARNISH:

roughly torn coriander leaves

1 First make the dressing. Chop the shallot very finely and place in a bowl with the fromage frais and cider vinegar. Mix well, season with salt and pepper to taste and set aside.

2 Peel the mangoes and cut the flesh either side of the stone to remove it. Thinly slice the mangoes.

3 Scatter the salad leaves decoratively on large, individual plates and arrange the mango slices prettily amongst them. Place the prawns on top. Using a teaspoon, drizzle the dressing over the salad. Serve garnished with coriander.

original

Sin-free

green

5½ Sins

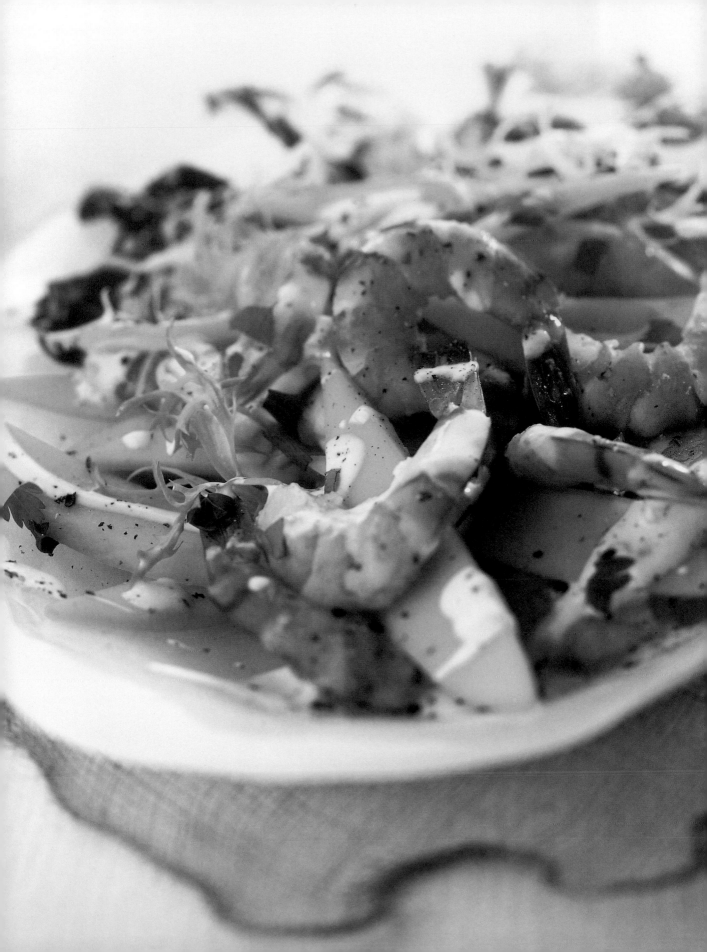

Tuna and mixed bean salad

Packed with robust flavours, this hearty salad combines fresh green beans and canned butter beans with chunks of tuna, in a piquant dressing. Serve this nutritious dish as a lunch or light supper.

serves **4**

preparation
10 minutes

cooking time
about 3 minutes

200g/7oz green beans, trimmed and halved

400g/14oz can butter beans, drained

200g/7oz can tuna chunks in brine, drained

1 red onion, peeled, halved and thinly sliced

3 tbsp chopped flat-leaf parsley

30g/1oz mixed salad leaves

FOR THE DRESSING:

juice of ½ lemon

2 tbsp fat-free French-style dressing

1 tsp mustard powder

salt and freshly ground black pepper

1 Add the green beans to a large pan of rapidly boiling water and cook for 2–3 minutes. Drain, refresh in cold water and place in a large bowl.

2 Rinse the butter beans under cold water, drain thoroughly and add to the green beans. Flake the tuna into large chunks and add to the beans with the red onion, chopped parsley and salad leaves.

3 To make the dressing, combine the lemon juice, French-style dressing and mustard in a small bowl and whisk until smooth. Season with salt and pepper.

4 Pour the dressing over the salad and toss gently to mix. Divide between large, individual plates and serve immediately.

Cook's note
You can use canned red salmon as an alternative to the tuna.

original

5½ Sins

green

2½ Sins

Aromatic Thai beef salad

Strips of juicy, rare beef and assorted crunchy fresh vegetables are tossed together with fragrant oriental flavourings of lemongrass, lime and pungent herbs for this delicious main course salad.

serves **4**

preparation
15 minutes

cooking time
about 3 minutes

450g/1lb lean beef steak, trimmed of
  visible fat
350g/12oz crisp Romaine or Cos lettuce
1 cucumber
2 carrots, peeled
100g/3½oz beansprouts
1 lemongrass stalk
small bunch of coriander

small bunch of Thai sweet basil
small bunch of mint
2 tsp sunflower oil
1 garlic clove, peeled and finely grated
juice of 2 limes
1 tbsp sweet chilli sauce
1 tbsp dark soya sauce
1 tbsp fish sauce

1 Thinly slice the beef and set aside. Finely shred the lettuce. Peel and dice the cucumber. Finely shred the carrots using a mandolin, or coarse grater. Rinse and drain the bean sprouts. Arrange the prepared vegetables on a large, shallow serving dish.

2 Discard the outer leaves from the lemongrass, then chop finely (to give you about 1 tablespoon). Strip the herb leaves from their stems and finely chop.

3 Heat the oil in a large, non-stick frying pan. When hot, add the garlic, lemongrass and beef. Stir-fry over a very high heat for 1–2 minutes, stirring continuously to separate the beef strips. Remove the meat from the pan with a slotted spoon and place on top of the prepared vegetables.

4 Add the lime juice to the pan with the chopped herbs. Add the sweet chilli, soya and fish sauces, and cook, stirring, for 30 seconds. Pour this dressing over the beef salad, toss to mix and serve immediately.

original

1 Sin

green

9 Sins

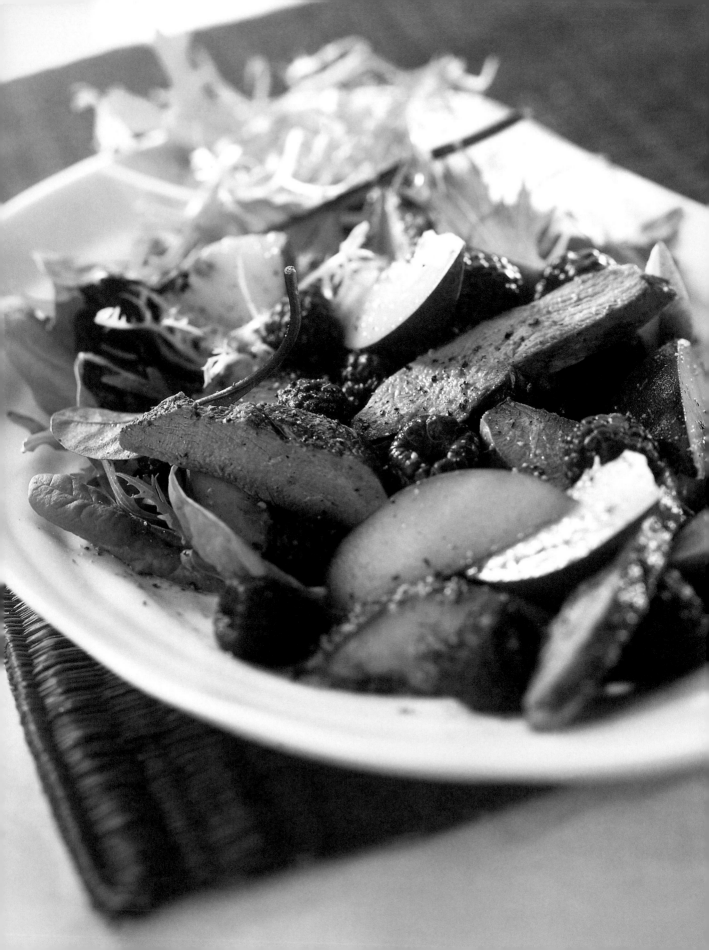

Duck, raspberry and peach salad

Juicy, red raspberries and succulent golden peaches combine with sliced, grilled duck breast to make a smart, original light lunch or supper.

2 boneless duck breasts, about 400g/14oz
   in total
salt and freshly ground black pepper
3 ripe peaches or nectarines
200g/7oz raspberries
60g/2oz mixed salad leaves

FOR THE DRESSING:
1 tbsp raspberry wine vinegar
1 tsp wholegrain mustard
1 tsp granulated artificial sweetener
salt and freshly ground black pepper

serves **4**
preparation
10 minutes
cooking time
about 14 minutes

1 Remove the skin and all visible fat from the duck breasts. Wash and pat dry with kitchen paper, then season and set aside.

2 Heat a ridged griddle pan over a high heat. When hot, place the duck breasts on the pan and cook for 6–7 minutes on each side. Remove from the heat, cover with foil and set aside to rest.

3 Meanwhile, halve, stone and slice the peaches or nectarines. Place in a bowl with the raspberries and mix gently. Set aside.

4 Make the dressing in another small bowl. Mix together the raspberry vinegar, wholegrain mustard and sweetener. Season with salt and pepper.

5 Thinly slice the duck breasts and gently mix with the fruit. Pour over the dressing and toss to mix. Arrange the salad leaves on large, individual plates and top with the salad. Serve immediately.

Cook's note
You can use chicken breasts as an alternative to the duck.

original

negligible

green

7 Sins

Citrus chicken salad

This mouth-watering salad, with its tangy, sweet flavours and creamy mustard and herb dressing, is perfect for a light, invigorating lunch or supper.

serves 4

preparation
10 minutes

cooking time
16–20 minutes

4 skinless, boneless chicken breasts, each
    about 150g/5oz
Fry Light for spraying
salt and freshly ground black pepper
1 large orange
1 small ruby grapefruit
15 red radishes, trimmed
1 red onion, peeled and halved
30g/1oz rocket leaves

FOR THE DRESSING:
4 tbsp chopped flat-leaf parsley
2 tbsp chopped fresh dill
2 tsp mustard powder
200g/7oz very low fat natural yogurt

1 Preheat the grill. Place the chicken on the grill pan and lightly spray with Fry Light. Season and cook under the hot grill for 8–10 minutes on each side or until cooked through.

2 While the chicken is cooking, prepare the salad ingredients. Cut the peel and all white pith from the orange and grapefruit, then carefully cut out the segments with a sharp knife and place in a bowl. Finely slice the radishes and red onion, then add to the fruit with the rocket leaves. Toss to mix.

3 To make the dressing, put the ingredients in a food processor and blend until smooth. Season with salt and pepper.

4 Cut the chicken into bite sized chunks and add to the salad. Pour over the dressing, toss to mix and serve immediately.

original

Sin-free

green

7½ Sins

Grilled chicken and red onion salad

For this light, flavoursome salad, you will need to allow a little time for the chicken to marinate before grilling. An aromatic balsamic, lemon and basil dressing is the perfect foil for grilled chicken and caramelised onion rings.

4 skinless, boneless chicken breasts, each
    about 150g/5oz

juice of 2 lemons

3 tbsp dark soya sauce

3 garlic cloves, peeled and crushed

freshly ground black pepper

1 red onion, peeled and sliced into rings

Fry Light for spraying

100g/3½oz mixed Italian-style salad leaves

1 ripe plum tomato, finely chopped

FOR THE DRESSING:

juice of 1 lemon

5 tbsp balsamic vinegar

2 garlic cloves, peeled and finely grated

5 tbsp chopped fresh basil leaves

salt and freshly ground black pepper

serves 4

preparation
10 minutes, plus marinating

cooking time
10 minutes

1 Cut the chicken into thin strips. Mix the lemon juice, soya sauce, garlic and some pepper together in a large bowl. Add the chicken, toss to mix, cover and leave to marinate in a cool place for 30 minutes.

2 Preheat the grill. Remove the chicken from the marinade and place on the grill pan with the onion rings. Spray lightly with Fry Light and grill for 10 minutes, turning the chicken and onion rings halfway through cooking.

3 Meanwhile, to make the dressing, place all the ingredients in a food processor and blend until smooth.

4 To serve, arrange the salad leaves on individual plates. Top with the grilled chicken strips and onion rings, then spoon over the dressing. Scatter with the chopped tomato and serve immediately.

original

Sin-free

green

7½ Sins

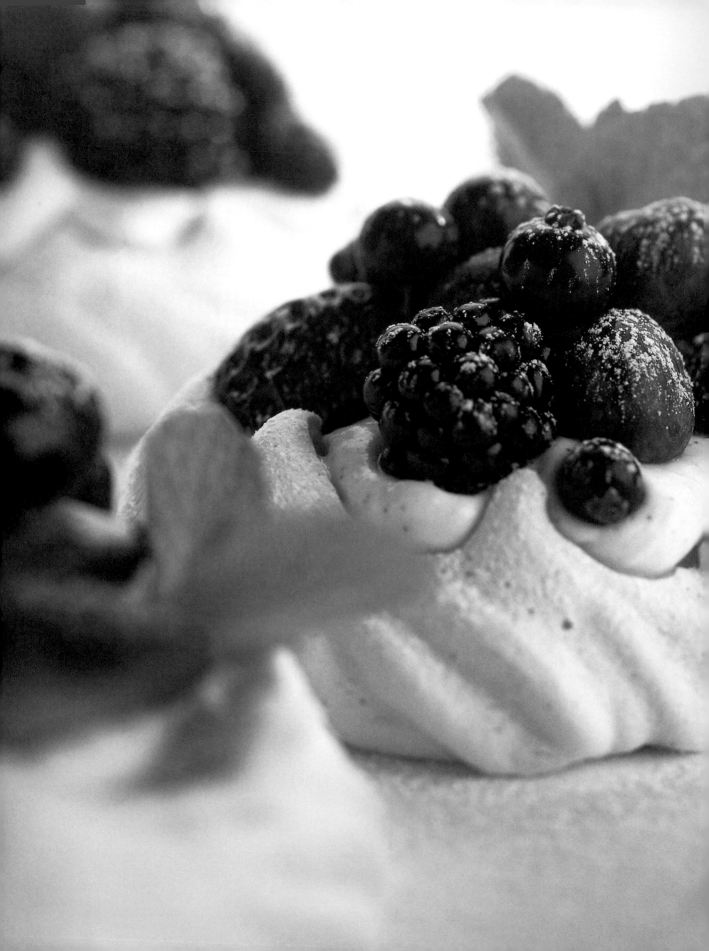

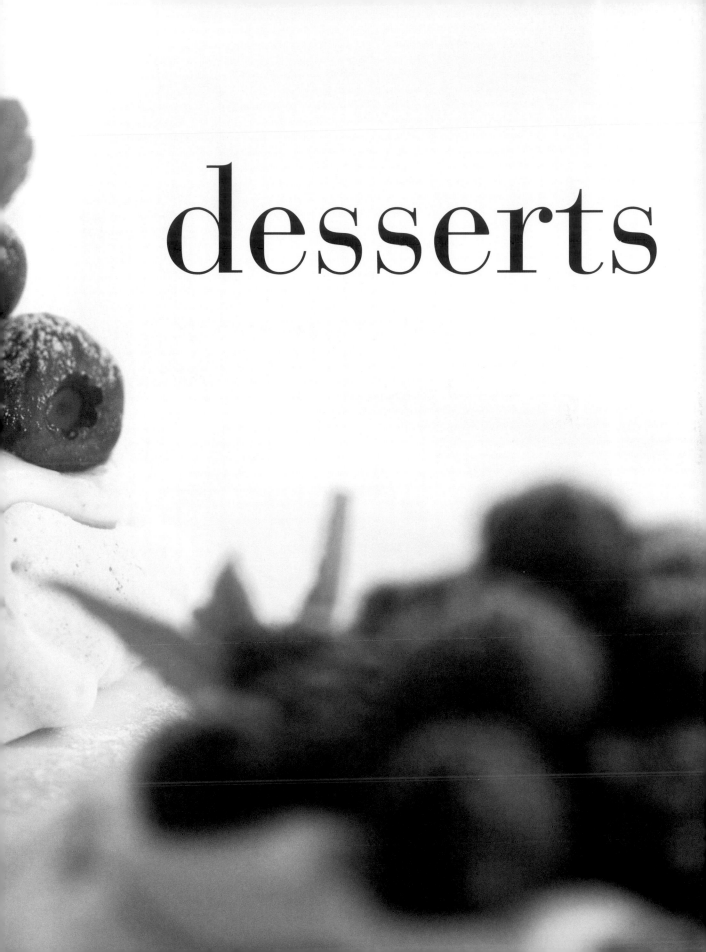

desserts

Mango and mint ice

A flavourful, fresh-tasting frozen yogurt ice, scented with juicy, tropical mango and fresh mint. Serve in small scoops, with slices of fresh mango and a scattering of mint leaves, for an elegant dessert.

serves **4**

preparation

10 minutes, plus freezing

✓ vegetarian

2 large, ripe mangoes

300g/10oz very low fat natural yogurt

2 tbsp chopped fresh mint leaves

1 tsp lime juice

TO SERVE:

1 large, ripe mango, peeled and thinly sliced

mint leaves to decorate

1 Peel the mangoes and cut the flesh away from the stone. Roughly chop the mango flesh and place in a food processor.

2 Add the yogurt, chopped mint and lime juice, and blend until very smooth. Transfer to a shallow, rigid freezerproof container, cover tightly and freeze for 3–4 hours.

3 Remove the semi-frozen mixture from the freezer and beat well with a fork to break down the ice crystals. Return to the freezer and freeze until firm.

4 Remove the sorbet from the freezer 15 minutes before serving. Scoop into glasses, bowls or dessert plates. Serve immediately, topped with mango slices and mint leaves.

original

4 Sins

green

4 Sins

Passion fruit and orange frozen yogurt

Ripe passion fruit lend their wonderful fragrance and depth of flavour to this refreshing iced dessert … the perfect tonic for a hot summer's day.

10 passion fruit

150ml/¼pt freshly squeezed orange juice

6 tbsp granulated artificial sweetener

250g/9oz very low fat natural yogurt

seeds and juice from 1 passion fruit to decorate

serves **4**

preparation

about 20 minutes, plus freezing

✓ vegetarian

1 Halve the passion fruit and scoop out the seeds and juice into a bowl, using a teaspoon.

2 Put the orange juice in a food processor with the sweetener and yogurt. Blend until smooth. Transfer to a shallow freezerproof container and fold in the passion fruit juice and seeds. Cover and freeze for 2 hours until slushy.

3 Remove the semi-frozen mixture from the freezer and beat well with a fork to break down the ice crystals. Return to the freezer for 30 minutes, then beat again. Repeat this process once more, then freeze for about 2 hours or until firm enough to scoop.

4 Remove the sorbet from the freezer about 20 minutes before serving to allow it to soften. Scoop into tall glasses and drizzle with passion fruit juice and seeds for a decorative finish.

original

1½ Sin

green

1½ Sin

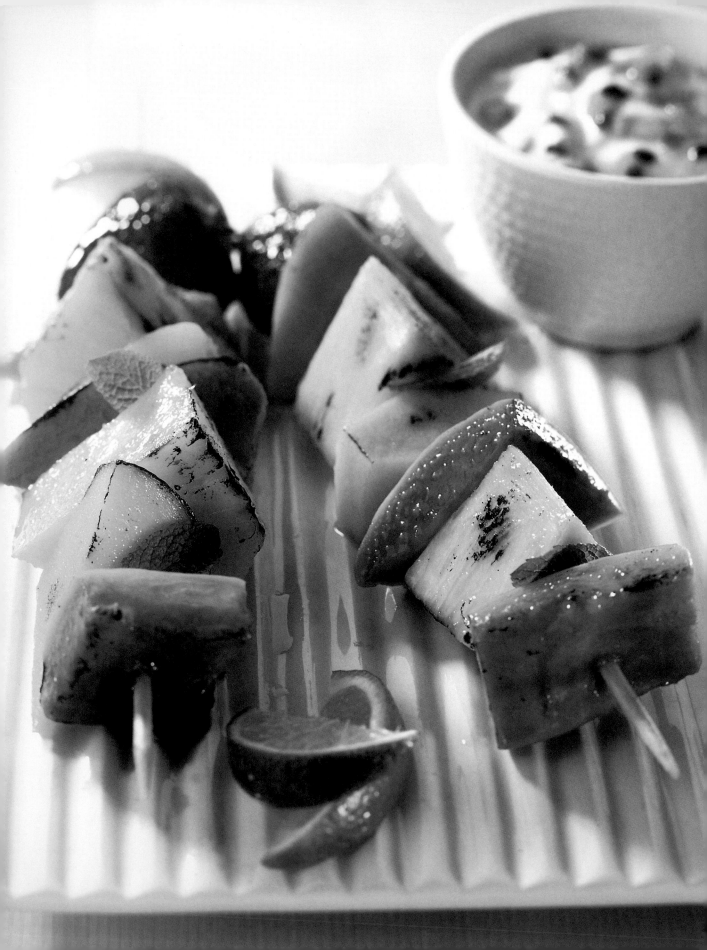

Grilled fruit skewers with passion fruit dip

Skewered tropical fruits and homegrown strawberries are grilled until lightly caramelised to make an unusual, easy dessert. A mouth-watering dip of passion fruit, honey and yogurt is the perfect accompaniment.

1 large mango

1 ripe papaya

¼ fresh pineapple

8 strawberries

juice of ½ lemon

1 tsp caster sugar

FOR THE DIP:

3 passion fruit

5 tbsp very low fat natural yogurt

1 tbsp honey

TO SERVE:

mint leaves (optional)

lime wedges

serves **4**

preparation

10 minutes

cooking time

5 minutes

✓ vegetarian

1 Peel the mango and cut the flesh away from the stone. Cut the papaya in half, scoop out the seeds and remove the peel. Peel and core the pineapple. Cut these tropical fruits into large chunks; leave the strawberries whole.

2 Preheat the grill. Thread the fruits alternately on to 8 pre-soaked wooden skewers and place the skewers on a grill pan. Sprinkle with the lemon juice and sugar. Place under the hot grill for 5 minutes, until the fruits are slightly caramelised, turning once.

3 Meanwhile, make the dip. Halve the passion fruit and scoop out the juice and seeds into a bowl. Add the yogurt and honey, and stir to mix.

4 Serve the skewers scattered with mint leaves, if you like. Accompany with the passion fruit dip and lime wedges.

Cook's note
It is important to soak the wooden skewers in warm water for about 20 minutes before use. This prevents them from scorching under the grill.

original

4½ Sins

green

4½ Sins

Caramelised oranges with redcurrants

A glossy caramelised orange. sprinkled with jewel-like redcurrants. is
a simple, refreshing way to round off a meal.

serves **4**

preparation
10 minutes,
plus chilling

cooking time
10 minutes

✓ vegetarian

4 seedless oranges

100g/3½oz caster sugar

120ml/4fl oz water

juice of 1 orange

100g/3½oz redcurrants

mint leaves to decorate (optional)

1 Thinly pare the zest from two of the oranges, using a swivel vegetable peeler,
then cut it into very thin strips. Add to a small pan of boiling water and
simmer for 5 minutes until softened. Drain and set aside.

2 Cut away all the pith and peel from the 4 oranges, using a sharp knife and
keeping the fruit whole. Place the oranges in a heatproof bowl and scatter the
blanched orange zest shreds over them.

3 Put the sugar, water and orange juice in a saucepan and dissolve over a low
heat. Bring to the boil and cook over a high heat until syrupy. Pour the syrup
over the oranges and leave to cool, then chill before serving.

4 To serve, place an orange on each serving plate and drizzle with some of the
syrup and orange zest strips. Sprinkle over the redcurrants and finish with
mint leaves if you like.

original

5 Sins

green

5 Sins

Hot rum banana flambé

Grilling bananas brings out their sweet, sunny flavour, and hot rum enhances this to delicious effect. Finish with a dusting of cinnamon for an easy, aromatic dessert that's served with a cooling dollop of fromage frais.

4 ripe bananas

1 tbsp light soft brown sugar

finely grated zest and juice of 1 lime

2 tbsp dark rum

1 tsp ground cinnamon

200g/7oz very low fat fromage frais

lime wedges to serve

1 Preheat the grill to high. Peel the bananas and cut them in half lengthways. Line a grill pan with foil and place the banana halves in the pan, cut side up.

2 Sprinkle the banana halves with the brown sugar and lime juice and cook under the hot grill for 3–4 minutes until they are golden brown and the sugar is melted and bubbling.

3 Meanwhile, pour the rum into a warmed, large metal ladle. Transfer the bananas to a warmed serving plate. Set the rum alight, using a long matchstick, and pour the flaming rum over the hot grilled bananas.

4 Scatter over the lime zest and dust the bananas with the cinnamon. Serve immediately, with the fromage frais and lime wedges on the side.

serves **4**

preparation

5 minutes

cooking time

3–4 minutes

✓ vegetarian

original

5½ Sins

green

5½ Sins

Pears poached in spiced red wine

Cinnamon, peppercorns and star anise add a zing to this aromatic variation of the classic French dessert. The poached pears are usually served chilled, but can be eaten warm if you prefer. For convenience, you can poach them a day in advance if you like.

serves **4**

preparation

10 minutes, plus optional chilling

cooking time

about 20 minutes

✓ vegetarian

4 ripe, dessert pears (Williams or Conference)

juice of 1 lemon

2 oranges

1 cinnamon stick

4–5 whole black peppercorns

2 star anise

2–3 cloves

150ml/¼pt red wine

150ml/¼pt diluted, no added sugar, blackcurrant cordial

3–4 tbsp granulated artificial sweetener

200g/7oz raspberries or blackberries

very low fat fromage frais, to serve

1 Peel the pears, leaving the stalks intact, and place in a bowl. Sprinkle the pears with the lemon juice (to prevent them from discolouring). Pare a few thin strips of zest from one of the oranges, using a swivel vegetable peeler.

2 Stand the pears in a saucepan, in which they fit fairly snugly. Add the orange zest strips, cinnamon, peppercorns, star anise and cloves. Pour in the wine and diluted blackcurrant cordial. Sprinkle over the sweetener. Bring to the boil, cover and cook on a medium heat for 10–15 minutes until the pears are just tender.

3 Meanwhile, slice off the top and bottom from the oranges using a sharp knife, then cut away the peel and pith. Cut each orange horizontally into 8 slices and place on a shallow serving dish, stacking the slices in pairs.

4 Remove the pears from the syrup and stand them on the orange slices. Boil the syrup rapidly for 4–5 minutes until slightly reduced and thickened.

5 Scatter the berries around the pears, then strain the reduced syrup over the fruit. Chill lightly before serving, or serve straight away if you prefer, accompanied by low fat natural fromage frais.

original

4 Sins

green

4 Sins

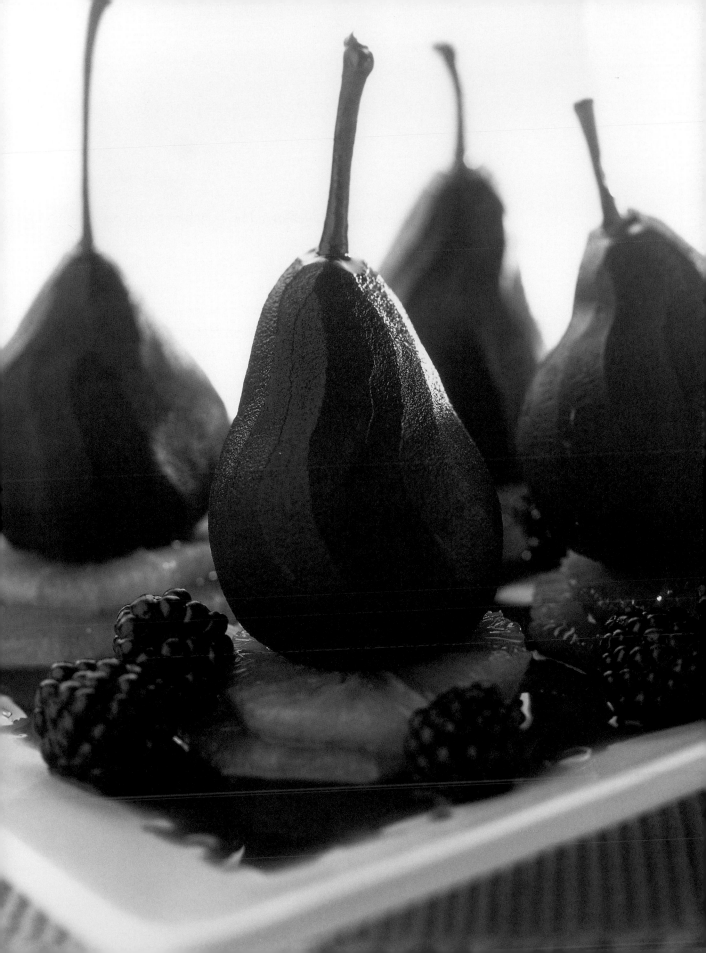

Poached figs with cinnamon cream

Poaching fresh figs gently in a light coffee and vanilla scented syrup brings out their wonderful flavour. A dollop of cinnamon flavoured 'cream' enhances the taste to delicious effect.

serves **4**

preparation

10 minutes,

plus standing

cooking time

about 10 minutes

✓ vegetarian

6 just-ripe figs
FOR THE POACHING LIQUID:
400ml/14fl oz lightly brewed coffee
5 tbsp clear honey
1 vanilla pod

FOR THE CINNAMON CREAM:
200g/7oz very low fat natural yogurt
1 tsp ground cinnamon
1 tsp granulated artificial sweetener
TO DECORATE:
mint leaves

1 For the poaching liquid, put the coffee and honey in a non-stick saucepan, large enough to hold the figs in a single layer. Split the vanilla pod in half lengthways and scrape out the seeds, using a small sharp knife, adding them to the pan with the empty pod. Bring to the boil and boil rapidly for 4–5 minutes. Turn off the heat.

2 Pierce the figs in several places with a fine, sharp skewer, then cut each one in half vertically. Place the fig halves in the poaching liquid in a single layer. Bring to a simmer over a moderate heat, cover and cook gently for 5–6 minutes.

3 Using a slotted spoon, transfer the figs to a serving bowl and set aside to cool. Strain the syrup over the figs and leave to stand at room temperature for 1 hour, to allow the flavours to infuse.

4 Meanwhile, make the cinnamon cream. Mix the ingredients together in a bowl, cover and chill until ready to serve.

5 To serve, place 3 fig halves in each individual, shallow serving bowl and spoon over the poaching syrup. Place a dollop of cinnamon cream on the side and top with a sprig of mint.

original

3½ Sins

green

3½ Sins

Italian-style amaretti stuffed peaches

This is a brilliant way to serve peaches at the height of their season. You simply stuff ripe peach halves with crushed almond biscuits mixed with soft cheese and almond liqueur, grill until bubbling, then serve with a dollop of creamy fromage frais.

4 large, ripe peaches

6 amaretti biscuits

1 egg yolk

1 tbsp golden caster sugar

60g/2oz Quark skimmed milk soft cheese

2 tbsp amaretto liqueur

juice of 1 small lemon

TO SERVE:

very low fat natural fromage frais

ground cinnamon and icing sugar to dust

serves **4**

preparation
10 minutes

cooking time
about 5 minutes

✓ vegetarian

1 Carefully cut the peaches in half and remove the stones. With a small sharp teaspoon, hollow out the flesh slightly to enlarge the stone cavity. Finely chop the scooped-out flesh and set aside in a bowl.

2 Place the amaretti biscuits in a clean, strong polythene bag and roughly crush with a rolling pin. Mix the crushed biscuits with the reserved peach flesh. Add the egg yolk, caster sugar, soft cheese and liqueur, and stir to mix well.

3 Preheat the grill to high. Place the peaches on a foil-lined grill pan, cut side up. Carefully spoon the amaretti stuffing into the peach cavities and sprinkle with the lemon juice. Place the peaches under the hot grill for about 5 minutes until the filling starts to bubble and brown.

4 To serve, place 2 peach halves on each serving plate and add a dollop of fromage frais. Lightly dust with cinnamon mixed with a pinch of icing sugar.

original

5½ Sins

green

5½ Sins

Summer berry cheesecake

This pretty, blueberry topped cheesecake isn't as sinful as it looks! The creamy filling of soft cheese and yogurt, with a zesty hint of lemon, is dotted with fresh strawberries and set on a crunchy gingernut biscuit base.

serves **6–8**

preparation
about 20 minutes, plus chilling

✓ vegetarian (see cook's note)

12 gingernut biscuits

30g/1oz low fat spread

4 tbsp cold water

2 x 11g/⅓oz sachets powdered gelatine

2 egg whites

2 x 250g/9oz pots Quark skimmed milk soft cheese

400g/14oz very low fat natural yogurt

finely grated zest of 1 small lemon

2 tbsp granulated artificial sweetener

100g/3½oz strawberries, hulled and finely chopped

200g/7oz blueberries

TO SERVE:

mint sprigs

pinch of icing sugar to dust (optional)

1 Line a 16cm/6½in springform cake tin with baking parchment. Place the biscuits in a clean, strong polythene bag and finely crush, using a rolling pin. Alternatively, crush in a food processor. Melt the low fat spread, add the biscuit crumbs and mix well. Spoon the mixture evenly over the prepared tin, then chill.

2 Put the water in a heatproof bowl, sprinkle the gelatine over, and leave to soften for a few minutes. Stand the bowl in a larger bowl containing boiling water and stir until the gelatine has dissolved. Leave to cool.

3 Whisk the egg whites until just stiff. Put the Quark, yogurt, lemon zest and sweetener in another bowl and stir until smooth. Stir the dissolved gelatine into the cheese mix, then fold in the whisked egg whites and strawberries. Pour this filling over the cheesecake base, cover and chill for about 3 hours until set.

4 When ready to serve, carefully release the cheesecake from the tin and arrange the blueberries on top. Serve cut into thin wedges, with a mint sprig on the side. Finish with a light dusting of icing sugar if you like.

original

4½–6 Sins

green

4½–6 Sins

Cook's note
For a vegetarian option, use vegi-gel, rather than gelatine.

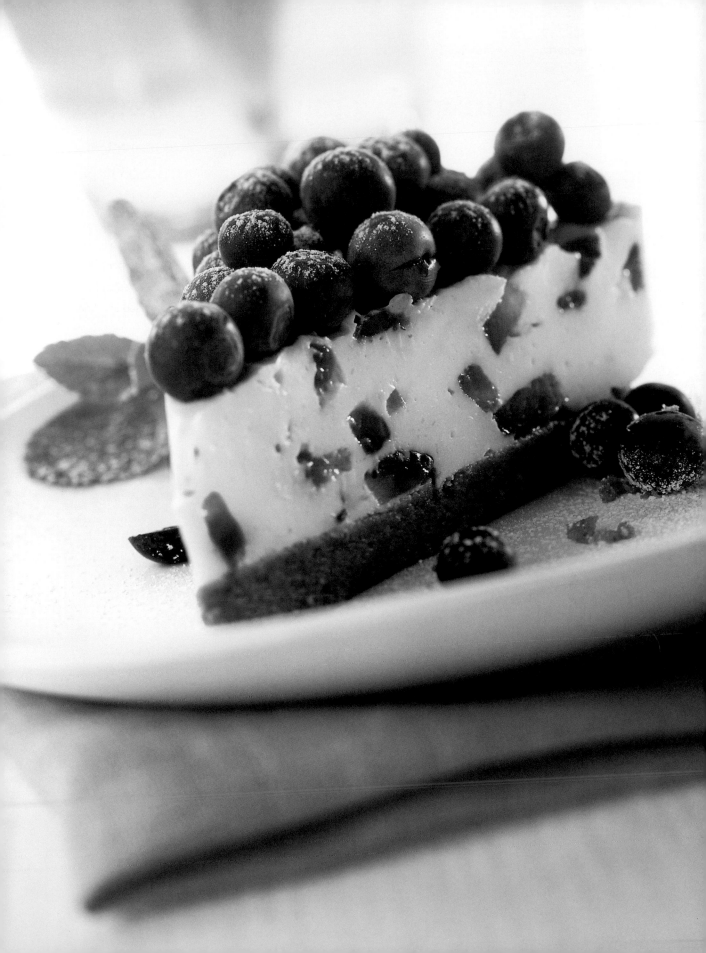

Strawberry zabaglione

A light, airy mixture of eggs, sugar and Marsala is fluffed up over a gentle heat, then spooned over flavourful strawberries. Serve while still warm for an instant dessert, or prepare ahead and chill before serving if you prefer.

serves **4**

preparation
5 minutes

cooking time
about 10–12
minutes

✓ vegetarian

200g/7oz strawberries, hulled

4 egg yolks

1 tsp vanilla essence

5 tbsp golden caster sugar

120ml/4fl oz Marsala

TO DECORATE:

sliced strawberries

mint leaves

1 Chop the strawberries into small pieces and divide them equally between 4 tall dessert glasses.

2 Put the egg yolks in the top of a double boiler, or in a heatproof bowl over a small saucepan of gently simmering water. The water should not touch the bottom of the bowl.

3 Add the vanilla essence, sugar and Marsala to the egg yolks and whisk (preferably using a hand-held electric whisk) for 10–12 minutes or until the mixture is pale, thick and warm. Make sure that the water is gently simmering under the bowl as you whisk.

4 When the zabaglione mixture is thick and creamy, spoon it over the strawberries in the dessert glasses. Serve immediately, topped with strawberry slices and mint leaves. Alternatively, you can cool and chill the dessert before serving.

original

6 Sins

green

6 Sins

Mango brûlée

Voluptuous, juicy orange mangoes snuggle beneath a creamy, vanilla flavoured topping. A grilled sugar crust provides the finishing touch.

1 large, ripe mango

150g/5oz very low fat Greek yogurt

1 tbsp vanilla essence

2 tsp granulated artificial sweetener

4 tbsp caster sugar

1 Peel the mango and cut the flesh away from the stone, then finely chop it and place in a bowl. Using a fork, lightly mash the mango flesh to a rough pulp.

2 Place 4 ramekins on a baking sheet. Divide the mango pulp between them and spread evenly.

3 Mix the yogurt, vanilla essence and artificial sweetener together in a bowl, then spoon the mixture over the mango in the ramekins. Level the surface and dust with the caster sugar.

4 Preheat the grill to its highest setting, then place the ramekins under the grill for 5 minutes or until the sugar topping is caramelised and golden. Alternatively, wave a cook's blow-torch over the surface of each dessert to caramelise the sugar. Allow to cool before serving.

serves **4**

preparation

10 minutes

cooking time

5 minutes,

plus cooling

✓ vegetarian

original

4½ Sins

green

4½ Sins

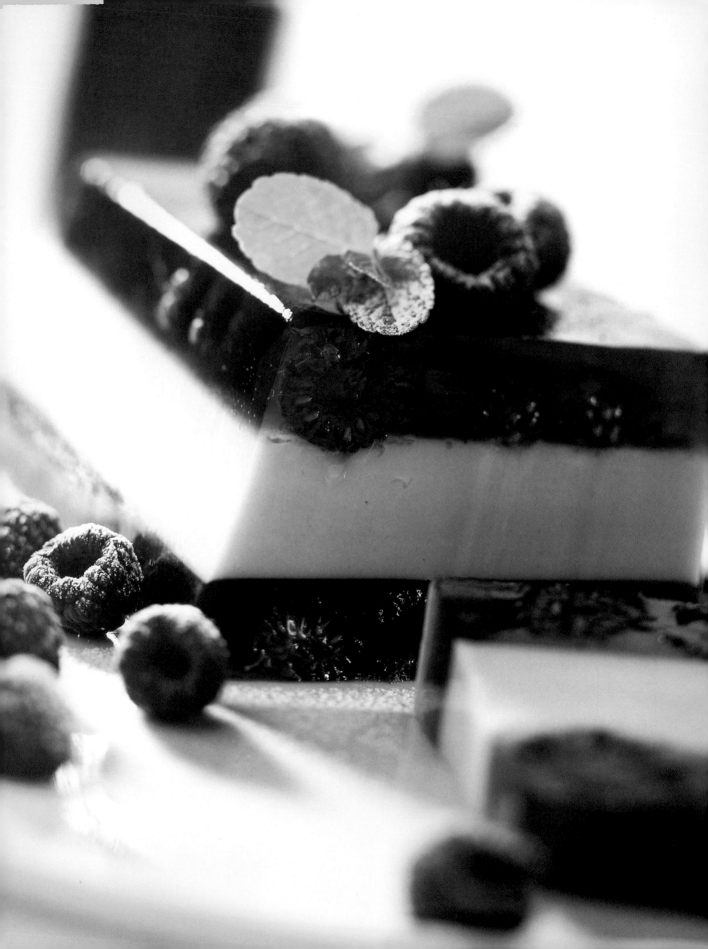

Raspberry and vanilla terrine

This impressive, mouth-watering dessert is easier to make than it looks and tastes sensational. To ring the changes, use strawberries in place of raspberries.

2 x 12g/½oz packets sugar-free raspberry
   jelly crystals
140ml/¼pt boiling water
2 tsp powdered gelatine
425ml/¾pt cold water
340g/12oz raspberries
225g/8oz very low fat fromage frais
1 tsp vanilla essence

TO DECORATE:
raspberries
mint sprigs
pinch of icing sugar to dust (optional)

serves **4**

preparation
15 minutes,
plus chilling

1 Place a 900g/2lb non-stick loaf tin in the freezer to chill. Place the jelly crystals in a heatproof jug and pour over the boiling water. Sprinkle in the gelatine and stir until dissolved, then top up with the cold water.

2 Cover the base of the loaf tin with a layer of raspberries. Pour in a quarter of the liquid jelly, then place the tin in the freezer for 10 minutes until set.

3 Combine the fromage frais and vanilla essence in a bowl and stir in half of the remaining liquid jelly. Spoon this mixture over the set raspberry jelly and refrigerate for about 30 minutes until set.

4 Arrange the remaining raspberries over the set fromage frais mixture and pour over the rest of the liquid jelly. Refrigerate for 2–3 hours until completely set.

5 When ready to serve, fill a basin or sink with hot water and dip the loaf tin in the water for 5–10 seconds to loosen the mould. Carefully invert on to a board or platter and shake gently to release the terrine. Top with raspberries and mint, and dust with a pinch of icing sugar if you wish. Serve cut into thick slices.

original
1 Sin

green
1 Sin

Espresso jellies

Quickly prepared in advance and chilled to set, these sparkling jellies make a light, refreshing end to a meal.

serves **4**

preparation

5 minutes, plus

chilling

✓ vegetarian (see

cook's note)

5 tbsp cold water

2 x 12g/⅓oz sachets powdered gelatine

600ml/1 pint hot brewed black coffee

4 tbsp golden caster sugar

TO SERVE:

cocoa powder to dust

very low fat natural fromage frais

1 Put the cold water in a large bowl, sprinkle the gelatine over the surface and leave to soak for 2–3 minutes. Add the hot black coffee and sugar, and stir well to dissolve the gelatine. Allow to cool.

2 Pour the coffee mixture into four 150ml/¼pt dariole moulds or ramekins. Stand on a small tray and place in the fridge for 3–4 hours until set.

3 When ready to serve, one at a time, dip the moulds or ramekins into a basin of hot water for 2–3 seconds, then carefully invert on to individual serving plates to unmould. Lightly dust the plate with cocoa powder and serve the jellies with fromage frais.

Cook's note

For a vegetarian option, use vegi-gel, which is derived from agar-agar (obtained from seaweed), rather than ordinary gelatine.

original

3 Sins

green

3 Sins

Mocha amaretto mousse

Surprisingly, this wicked creamy chocolate and coffee dessert is relatively low in Sins. Spiked with almond flavoured liqueur to enhance the mocha flavour, it tastes superb.

60g/2oz good quality dark chocolate
    (minimum 70% cocoa solids)
2 tsp instant coffee granules
2 tbsp amaretto liqueur
1 tbsp water

3 eggs, separated
200g/7oz Quark skimmed milk soft cheese
2 tbsp granulated artificial sweetener
mint leaves to decorate (optional)

serves **4**

preparation

15 minutes, plus chilling

✓ vegetarian

1 Break the chocolate into small pieces and place in a heatproof bowl over a pan of gently simmering water, making sure the bowl does not touch the water. Add the instant coffee, liqueur and 1tbsp water. Stir until the chocolate has melted, the coffee is dissolved and the mixture is smooth. Set aside to cool.

2 Meanwhile, place the egg yolks in a large bowl with the Quark and sweetener and whisk thoroughly until thick and pale. Fold in the cooled chocolate mixture and set aside.

3 Whisk the egg whites in a clean, large bowl until softly peaking. Using a large metal spoon, carefully fold them into the chocolate mixture until smoothly incorporated. Divide between 4 individual serving bowls and refrigerate for 2–3 hours until set. Serve chilled, topped with mint leaves if desired.

original

4½ Sins

green

4½ Sins

Rum and chocolate pots

Conveniently prepared in advance, this totally indulgent chocolate dessert is the perfect end to a dinner party. Fresh cherries and berries, fromage frais and a light dusting of cocoa provide a decadent finish.

serves **4**

preparation

20 minutes, plus chilling

✓ vegetarian

85g/3oz good quality dark, bitter plain
    chocolate (minimum 70% cocoa solids)
3 medium eggs, separated
4 tbsp granulated artificial sweetener
2 tbsp dark rum
100g/3½oz very low fat natural fromage frais

TO SERVE:
cocoa powder for dusting
cherries, strawberries and/or raspberries
tiny mint sprigs (optional)

1 Break the chocolate into small pieces and place in a heatproof bowl over a pan of gently simmering water, making sure the bowl does not touch the water. Leave until the chocolate has melted, stir until smooth and leave to cool for 10 minutes.

2 Beat the egg yolks in a bowl until pale and thick, then gradually beat in the sweetener and rum. Whisk the egg whites in a clean, large bowl until firm peaks form.

3 Fold the egg yolk mixture into the cooled chocolate, then carefully fold in the whisked egg whites using a large metal spoon. Spoon the mixture into 4 small pots, bowls or cups and chill for 2–3 hours until set.

4 When ready to serve, stir the fromage frais until smooth and place a spoonful on top of each chocolate 'pot'. Stand them on individual plates and decorate with fresh cherries and strawberries, or raspberries. Lightly dust with cocoa and finish with tiny mint sprigs if desired.

original

6 Sins

green

6 Sins

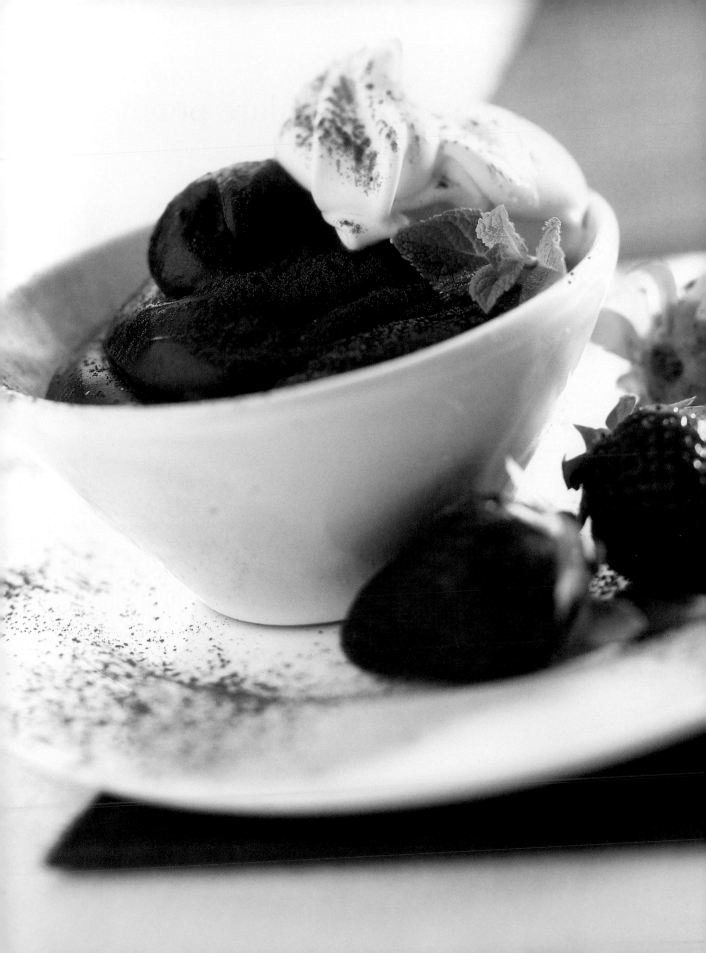

Chocolate and peach roulade

For this dreamy dessert, a moist chocolate sponge is rolled around a delectable filling of sweet, chopped peaches enveloped in creamy fromage frais.

serves **8**

preparation

20 minutes, plus chilling

cooking time

15–18 minutes

✓ vegetarian

6 eggs, separated

100g/3½oz caster sugar

6 tbsp granulated artificial sweetener

55g/2oz cocoa powder, sifted

200g/7oz very low fat natural fromage frais

200g/7oz canned peaches in natural juice, drained

TO SERVE:

fresh peach slices (optional)

icing sugar and cocoa to dust

1 Preheat the oven to 180°C/Gas 4. Line a 33 x 23cm/13 x 9in Swiss roll tin with baking parchment.

2 Whisk the egg yolks with the sugar and 4 tbsp of the sweetener in a large bowl until pale and thick. Carefully fold in the cocoa, using a large metal spoon.

3 Whisk the egg whites in a clean bowl until firm peaks form, then carefully fold in the cocoa mixture. Pour into the prepared tin and bake in the middle of the oven for 15–18 minutes until set and springy to the touch. Leave to cool in the tin.

4 Meanwhile, make the filling. Mix the fromage frais with the remaining sweetener in a bowl. Roughly chop the canned peaches and set aside.

5 Turn out the sponge on to a clean sheet of baking parchment and carefully peel off the lining paper. Spread the fromage frais over the sponge and scatter the chopped peaches on top. Lift one of the shorter ends of the paper and carefully roll up the sponge, using the paper to help. Do not worry if the sponge cracks slightly. Press gently to seal the edge.

6 Place the roulade on a serving plate, cover and chill for 30 minutes to 1 hour. To serve, dust lightly with icing sugar and cocoa, then cut into slices. Accompany with fresh peach slices if available.

original

4 Sins

green

4 Sins

Pineapple crush

Sweet, tropical pineapple is layered with crushed meringue and cinnamon flavoured fromage frais to create a light, refreshing dessert.

500g/1lb 2oz fresh, sweet, ripe pineapple

4–5 tbsp water

2 tbsp granulated artificial sweetener

4 ready-made individual meringue nests

350g/12oz very low fat natural fromage frais

1 tsp ground cinnamon

serves **4**

preparation

10 minutes,

plus chilling

cooking time

6–8 minutes

✓ vegetarian

1 Peel and core the pineapple, then cut into 2cm/¾in dice. Place in a small saucepan with the water and bring to the boil. Cover and simmer gently for 4–5 minutes.

2 Add the sweetener and mix thoroughly. Leave to cool completely, then cover and chill the pineapple mixture in the refrigerator for 1–2 hours.

3 To serve, place the meringue nests in a bowl and crush lightly. Mix the fromage frais with the ground cinnamon and lightly fold into the meringue mixture. Layer the crushed meringue mixture with the chilled pineapple in 4 dessert glasses or bowls. Serve immediately.

original

6 Sins

green

6 Sins

Summer berry pavlovas

This ultra-quick and easy version of the classic New Zealand dessert partners fresh, juicy summer berries with light, chewy meringues. It is perfect for an alfresco dinner party, and you can ring the changes by using chopped tropical fruit – mango, pineapple and papaya – rather than berries.

serves **4**

preparation

20 minutes

✓ vegetarian

200g/7oz small strawberries, hulled

100g/3½oz blackberries

100g/3½oz blueberries

40g/1½oz redcurrants

juice of 1 orange

200g/7oz very low fat fromage frais

1 vanilla pod

2 tsp granulated artificial sweetener

4 ready-made individual meringue nests

TO SERVE:

mint sprigs to decorate

icing sugar to dust

1 Cut any larger strawberries in half. Place half of them in a bowl with the blackberries, blueberries and redcurrants.

2 Put the remaining strawberries in a food processor with the orange juice and blend until smooth. Transfer to a bowl, cover and refrigerate.

3 Place the fromage frais in another bowl. Split the vanilla pod in half lengthways and scrape out the seeds, using a small sharp knife; add them to the fromage frais. Sprinkle in the sweetener and stir to mix well.

4 To serve, place the meringue nests on individual plates. Spoon the fromage frais mixture into the nests and pile the berries on top. Drizzle the strawberry and orange purée around the meringue nests and serve immediately, decorated with mint sprigs and a light dusting of icing sugar.

original

4½ Sins

green

4½ Sins

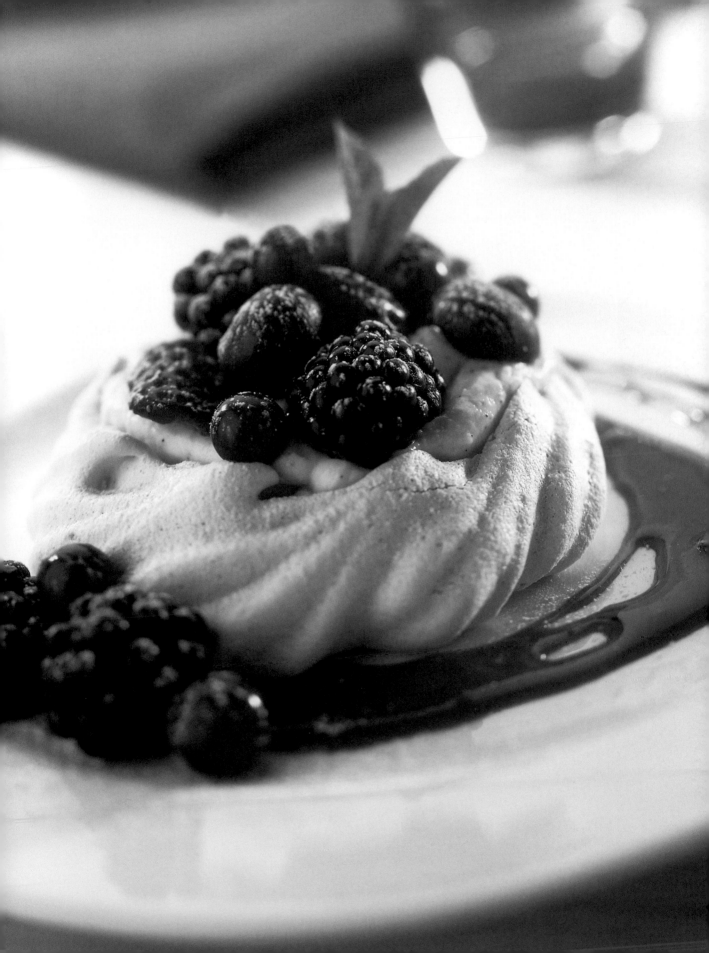

Individual lime meringue puddings

This tangy dessert is a variation of lemon meringue pie ... but without the high-fat pastry. For a lemony taste, simply substitute the limes with small lemons.

serves **4**

preparation and **cooking time**

25 minutes

✓ vegetarian

3 tbsp cornflour

150ml/¼pt cold water

finely grated zest and juice of 3 large limes

6 tbsp golden caster sugar

2 large eggs, separated

TO SERVE:

shredded lime zest to decorate

cocoa powder to dust

1 Preheat the oven to 200°C/Gas 6. Mix the cornflour and cold water together in a small saucepan until smooth. Add the lime zest and juice and slowly bring to the boil, stirring constantly. When the mixture starts to thicken, remove from the heat and stir in 4 tbsp of the sugar. Stir well and set aside to cool.

2 Lightly beat the egg yolks and stir into the cooled lime mixture. Spoon into 4 ramekins and place on a baking sheet. Cook in the oven for 5 minutes.

3 Meanwhile, whisk the egg whites in a large, clean bowl until stiff, but not dry. Gradually whisk in the remaining sugar, and continue to whisk until the meringue is stiff and glossy.

4 Spoon the meringue over the lime mixture in the ramekins, swirling it with a small palette knife to form peaks. Bake in the oven for 8–10 minutes, or until the meringue is lightly tinged brown.

5 Serve straight away, or allow to cool and chill lightly before serving. Scatter a little finely grated lime zest on top of the puddings and dust lightly with cocoa powder to finish.

original

7½ Sins

green

7½ Sins

Rhubarb and ginger crumble sundaes

This successful combination of flavours and contrasting textures comprises layers of tart rhubarb, mixed with sweetened spiced ginger, crushed gingernut biscuits and creamy fromage frais.

450g/1lb rhubarb, trimmed

5 tbsp water

1 tsp ground ginger

1 tsp mixed spice

4 tbsp granulated artificial sweetener

8 gingernut biscuits

200g/7oz very low fat natural fromage frais

mint leaves to decorate

1 Cut the rhubarb into 2.5cm/1in pieces and place in a medium saucepan with the water. Bring to the boil, cover and simmer for 8–10 minutes until tender. Allow to cool, then stir in the ground ginger, mixed spice and sweetener.

2 Place the ginger biscuits in a strong polythene bag and crush coarsely with a rolling pin or mallet. Put the fromage frais in a bowl and stir until smooth.

3 Layer the spiced, sweetened rhubarb with the crushed ginger biscuits and fromage frais in 4 dessert glasses or bowls. Serve immediately, or chill in the refrigerator for 1–2 hours before serving. Decorate with mint leaves.

serves **4**

preparation
10 minutes, plus cooling

cooking time
8–10 minutes

✓ vegetarian

original

5½ Sins

green

5½ Sins

reference

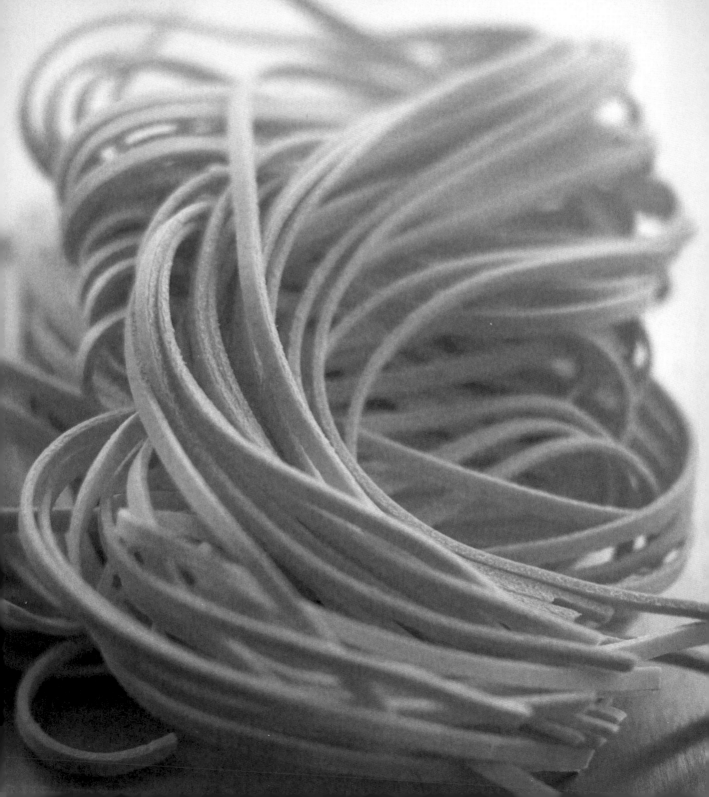

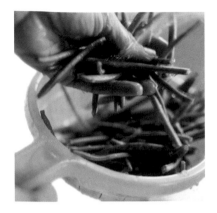
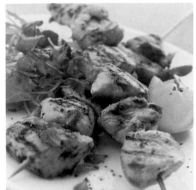
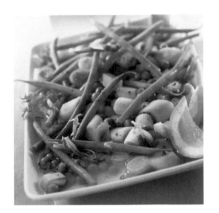
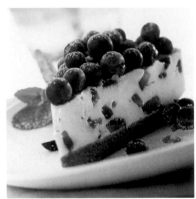
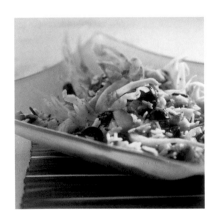
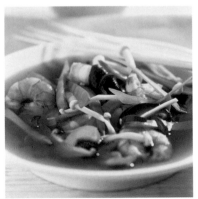
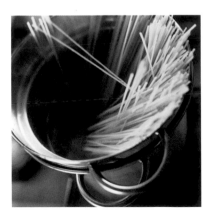

Recipe Sin Values

The Sins listed for each of the recipes in this book are per portion.

STARTERS	Page	Original	Green
Aubergine pâté with crudités	48	Sin-free	Sin-free
Tomato, garlic and basil bruschetta	49	7	7
Watermelon salad with feta dressing	51	1	1
Spinach and egg tartlets	52	3	3
Red pepper and potato frittata	53	2½	1½
Grilled vegetables with herb salsa	54	Sin-free	Sin-free
Stuffed portobello mushrooms	56	1	1
Italian-style mussels	57	2½	7½
Gravadlax with cucumber and watercress cream	58	negligible	6
Grilled seafood skewers	60	Sin-free	4½
Herbed tuna cream on lettuce leaves	61	negligible	2½
Spiced koftes with minted yogurt dip	62	1	7
Parma ham with minted melon wedges	64	Sin-free	4
Seared chicken livers on rocket leaves	65	2	8
Creamy gazpacho	67	Sin-free	Sin-free
Chinese mushroom and tofu soup	68	Sin-free	Sin-free
Corn and coriander chowder	69	7	1½
Thai prawn and lemongrass soup	70	Sin-free	2
Chunky fish soup	72	negligible	7½
Italian chicken and tomato soup	73	Sin-free	5

FISH	Page	Original	Green
Baltimore fish cakes	76	3½	9½
Spicy crab wedges	77	Sin-free	3½
Moroccan spiced fish kebabs	78	Sin-free	4
Creamy prawn curry	80	Sin-free	7½
Prawn and chive omelette	81	Sin-free	3
Griddled scallops with a herb dressing	83	1½	6
Griddled squid with Thai-style dressing	84	Sin-free	4½

	Page	Original	Green
Herby salmon and prawn pie	85	2	14½
Salmon with tropical fruit salsa	86	½	18
Steamed coconut and coriander salmon	88	½	18
Chinese-style steamed fish	89	½	10½
Seared tuna with hot pepper sauce	90	Sin-free	14
Charred chermoula mackerel with a citrus and olive salad	92	1	23
Baked red mullet with pesto	93	2½	13½
Grilled trout with dill mayonnaise	94	2	14
French fish stew	96	Sin-free	5½
Tandoori monkfish	97	Sin-free	5
Cod and vegetable parcels	99	1½	7½
Baked haddock with steamed oriental greens	100	1	5
Haddock and tomato roast	101	1½	8½

MEAT

	Page	Original	Green
Chicken and Parma ham saltimbocca	104	2½	15
Parchment chicken	105	½	11
Coriander and mint grilled chicken skewers	106	½	16
Chargrilled Caribbean chicken	108	Sin-free	12
Japanese-style chicken with vegetables	109	1	11½
Spanish-style chicken	111	2	9½
Herby mushroom and cheese turkey rolls	112	Sin-free	10½
Creamy turkey and mushroom ragoût	113	2	9
Grilled gammon steaks and tomatoes with herb mash	114	Sin-free	14
Honey, soy and ginger duck breasts	116	½	14½
Peppered venison steaks with a fruity mash	117	1½	10½
Chive and ginger pork stir-fry	118	½	8
Sweet pepper, pork and pineapple casserole	120	3	8½
Pork and apple burgers on a wilted spinach salad	121	1	11½
Chargrilled fillet steak with roasted vegetables	123	1½	13½
Pan-fried beef with herbs and balsamic vinegar	124	1½	17½
Creamy beef and mushroom stroganoff	125	3	10
Shish kebabs with kachumber	126	2	12
Spicy lamb steaks	128	Sin-free	10
Creamy lamb's liver with bacon and onions	129	2½	10½

VEGETARIAN	Page	Original	Green
Herb and sweet potato rosti	132	7	Sin-free
Oriental tofu omelettes	133	2½	1½
Spinach, pea and mint frittata	135	2½	1½
Bean and mushroom burgers	136	8½	Sin-free
Tex Mex chilli	137	11	½
Vegetable balti	138	2	negligible
Italian vegetable stew	140	8	½
Penne arrabiata (without Parmesan)	141	15	Sin-free
Linguini with spring greens, garlic and chilli	142	18	3
Spaghetti with courgette and cherry tomato sauce	144	16½	1½
Aubergine and pasta gratin	145	17	4½
Pappardelle primavera	146	16	1
Orange and ginger noodles	148	17	½
Vegetable chow mein	149	7	Sin-free
Roasted Mediterranean vegetable couscous	151	12½	½
Jewelled tabbouleh	152	7½	Sin-free
Cheesy vegetable and rice bake	153	10	4
Chilli and butternut squash risotto	154	13½	2
Mixed vegetable pilau rice	156	12	Sin-free
Special vegetable fried rice	157	12	Sin-free

VEGETABLES AND SALADS	Page	Original	Green
Stir-fried cabbage with spring greens	160	½	½
French-style ratatouille	161	negligible	negligible
Lime and lemon courgettes	162	1½	1½
Mixed mushrooms with garlic, lemon and parsley	164	Sin-free	Sin-free
Baked stuffed herbed tomatoes	165	Sin-free	Sin-free
Spring vegetable sauté with herbs	167	3	1½
Cajun-style vegetables	168	Sin-free	Sin-free
Creamy dal	169	12	Sin-free
Spiced roasted baby new potatoes	170	13	Sin-free
Boulangère potatoes	172	6½	negligible
Roasted asparagus with a balsamic dressing	173	Sin-free	Sin-free
Fennel and wild rice salad	174	8	½

	Page	Original	Green
Apple and baby spinach salad	176	1½	1½
Piquant crab salad	177	2	11
Prawn and mango salad	178	Sin-free	5½
Tuna and mixed bean salad	180	5½	2½
Aromatic Thai beef salad	181	1	9
Duck, raspberry and peach salad	183	negligible	7
Citrus chicken salad	184	Sin-free	7½
Grilled chicken and red onion salad	185	Sin-free	7½

DESSERTS	Page	Original	Green
Mango and mint ice	188	4	4
Passion fruit and orange frozen yogurt	189	1½	1½
Grilled fruit skewers with passion fruit dip	191	4½	4½
Caramelised oranges with redcurrants	192	5	5
Hot rum banana flambé	193	5½	5½
Pears poached in spiced red wine	194	4	4
Poached figs with cinnamon cream	196	3½	3½
Italian-style amaretti stuffed peaches	197	5½	5½
Summer berry cheesecake	198	4½–6	4½–6
Strawberry zabaglione	200	6	6
Mango brûlée	201	4½	4½
Raspberry and vanilla terrine	203	1	1
Espresso jellies	204	3	3
Mocha amaretto mousse	205	4½	4½
Rum and chocolate pots	206	6	6
Chocolate and peach roulade	208	4	4
Pineapple crush	209	6	6
Summer berry pavlovas	210	4½	4½
Individual lime meringue puddings	212	7½	7½
Rhubarb and ginger crumble sundaes	213	5½	5½

Free foods selection

- We have listed many of our Free Foods here. For the full list, you will need to become a Slimming World member.
- Foods with an S symbol will give your weight loss a boost. Choosing foods marked with an SS symbol will give your weight loss an even bigger boost.

- Foods marked with an F will give you extra fibre and those marked with FF will give you an even richer helping of fibre.
- Foods marked H will keep you healthy and those marked HH are vital to your health and a selection of these needs to be included every day.

GREEN CHOICE FREE FOODS

All vegetables are classed as a Free Food when on a Green day.

Potatoes			HH
Rice			H
Dried pasta			H
Buckwheat			H
Couscous			H
Baked beans	F	SS	H
Chick peas	F		H
Red kidney beans	FF	S	H
Soya beans	FF		H
Lentils	F	S	H
Peas	F	SS	H
Quorn	F	SS	H
Eggs			
Tofu			
Apples		S	HH
Bananas			HH
Grapefruit		SS	HH
Oranges		S	HH
Peaches		S	HH
Pineapple		S	HH
Strawberries		SS	HH
Very low fat natural yogurt			H
Very low fat natural fromage frais			H

ORIGINAL CHOICE FREE FOODS

Not all vegetables are Free Foods on the Original Choice: choose from only those listed here for a Sin-free day. All cuts of meat should be lean with all visible fat removed.

Artichokes	F	S	HH
Asparagus		S	HH
Aubergine		S	HH
Baby corn cobs		S	HH

Beans – French, runner	F	S	HH
Beetroot		S	HH
Broccoli	F	S	HH
Brussels sprouts	F	S	HH
Cabbage		S	HH
Carrots		S	HH
Cauliflower		S	HH
Courgettes		S	HH
Leeks		S	HH
Mushrooms		S	HH
Onions		S	HH
Spinach		S	HH
Squash		S	HH
Swede		S	HH
Quorn	F	SS	H
Chicken/turkey (fat and skin removed)			H
Cod/haddock/sole/plaice		SS	H
Kippers			H
Mackerel/pilchards			H
Salmon			H
Crab			H
Prawns		S	H
Bacon			
Beef			
Lamb			
Pork/ham			
Eggs			
Tofu			
Apples		S	HH
Bananas			HH
Grapes			HH
Oranges		S	HH
Pineapple		S	HH
Strawberries		SS	HH
Very low fat natural yogurt			H
Very low fat natural fromage frais			H

Healthy extras

The full Food Optimising system given to members at class also includes 'Healthy Extras', which ensure a good overall balance of nutrients in addition to those obtained from Free Foods, with particular emphasis on calcium and fibre-rich foods. They include dairy products, bread, crispbreads and cereals, as well as lean meats, poultry, fish, nuts and seeds (on the Green choice) and pasta, potatoes and pulses (on the Original choice).

'Sins' selection

Here is a selection of Sin values for foods which you can enjoy every day. A list of over 40,000 Sin values is available from Slimming World (see page 224).

ALCOHOL

30ml/1fl oz measure of any spirit	2½
150ml/¼ pt glass of wine	5
300ml/½ pt lager/beer	5
300ml/½ pt cider	5

BISCUITS AND BARS

Each unless otherwise stated

Custard cream	3
Digestive	4
Cheese thin	1
Chocolate finger	1½
Rich tea/marie	2
Jaffa cake/gingernut	2½
Shortcake	2½
Go Ahead Crispy Fruit Slices	3
Special K Cereal Bar	4½

CRISPS

Per standard bag

French Fries/Golden Lights	4½
Thai Bites	4½
Quavers	5
Wotsits	5½
Go Ahead Crinkled Potato Chips	6
Snack-a-Jacks, 30g/1oz bag	6
Standard potato crisps, per 30g/1oz	7½

CHOCOLATE AND SWEETS

Per standard bar/tube/bag unless otherwise stated

Fun-size bars	5
Two-finger Kit Kat	5½
Milkybar	3½
Penguin bar	7
Maltesers	9
Flake	9

CAKES

Individual, average

Custard tart	13
Jam doughnut	12½
Danish pastry	20½
Mince pie	11½
Eccles cake	10½
Mr Kipling Cake Bites	1½
Mr Kipling Country/Lemon Slices	6

DESSERTS

Müllerice, 99% fat free, per pot	5½
Müllerlight mousse, 99.9% fat free, per pot	7½

To enjoy any of the delicious desserts on pages 186–213, check the Sin value (listed alongside each recipe, and on pages 216–9) and count this into your daily allowance.

SAUCES AND SPREADS

Gravy made from granules, with no fat 4 level tbsp	1
Reduced calorie mayonnaise 1 level tbsp	2½
Custard made with slimmed milk 2 level tbsp	1
Margarine/spread, low fat variety 30g/1oz	5½
Olive oil/any oil 1 level tablespoon	6

NUTS

Almonds, shelled, 30g/1oz	8½
Brazil nuts, shelled, 30g/1oz	9½
Cashew nuts, shelled, 30g/1oz	8
Peanuts, fresh/roast, 30g/1oz	8½
Walnuts, shelled, 30g/1oz	9½

Index

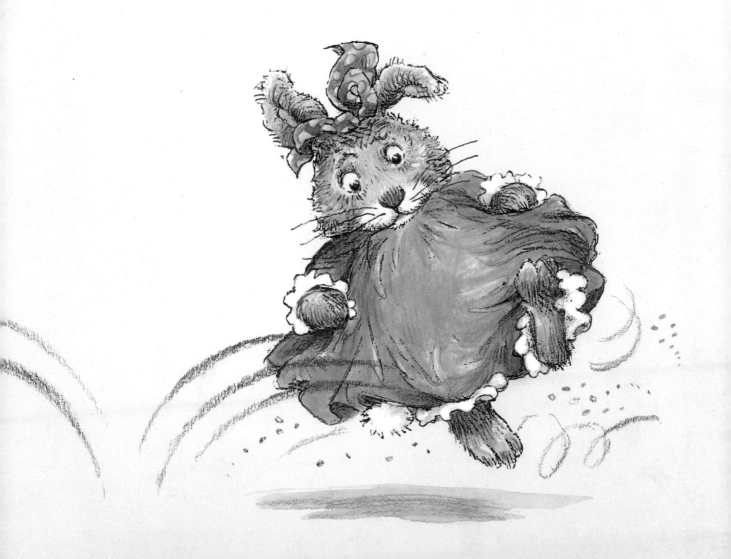

First published in the United Kingdom in 1999 by Ragged Bears Publishing Limited,
Milborne Wick, Sherborne, Dorset DT9 4PW

Distributed by Ragged Bears Limited, Ragged Appleshaw, Andover, Hampshire SP11 9HX
Tel: 01264 772269

A CIP record of this book is available from the British Library

ISBN 1 85714 193 8

Printed in Singapore

Hyacinth Hop has the Hic-Hops

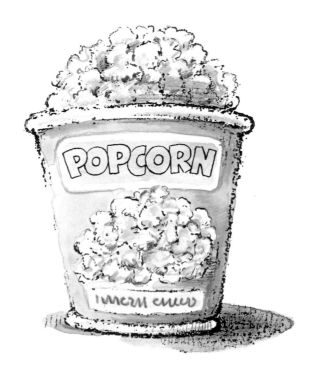

POPCORN

written and illustrated by

Tony Kenyon

Ragged Bears Publishing

"The popcorn's gone!" said Hyacinth's brother
Henry,

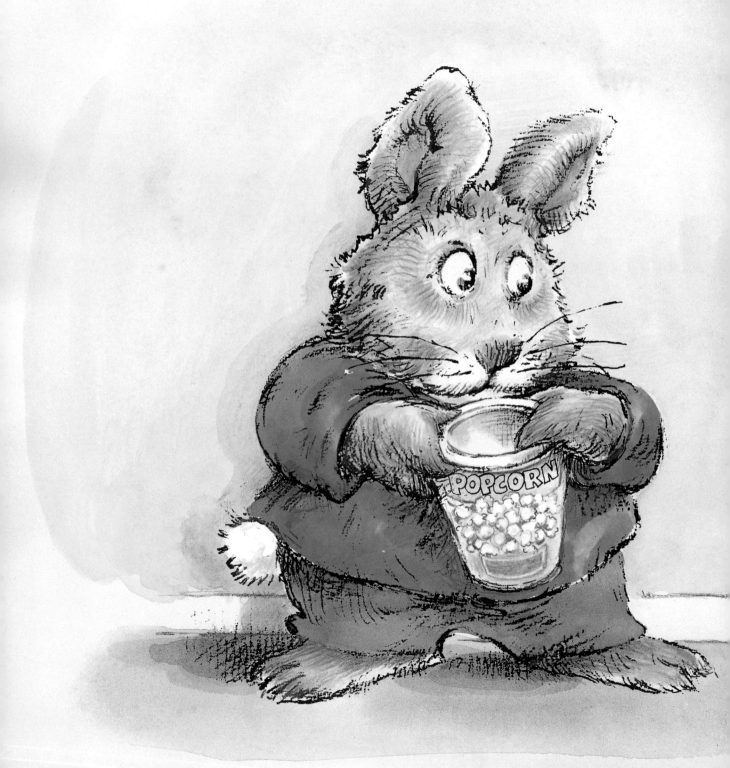

"Hyacinth Hop has eaten the lot and Hyacinth Hop has the hic-hops."

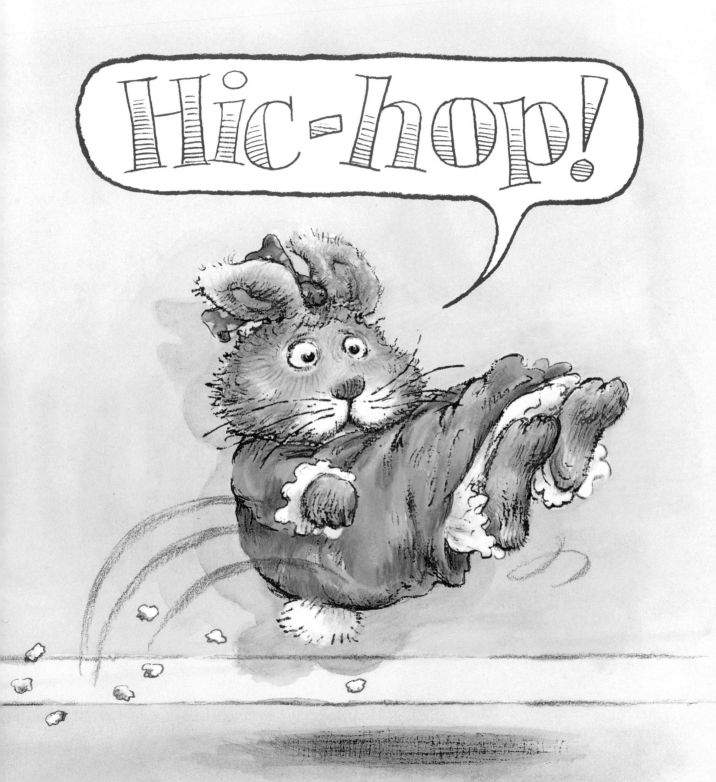

"A glass of water is a cure for hic-hops," said Henry.

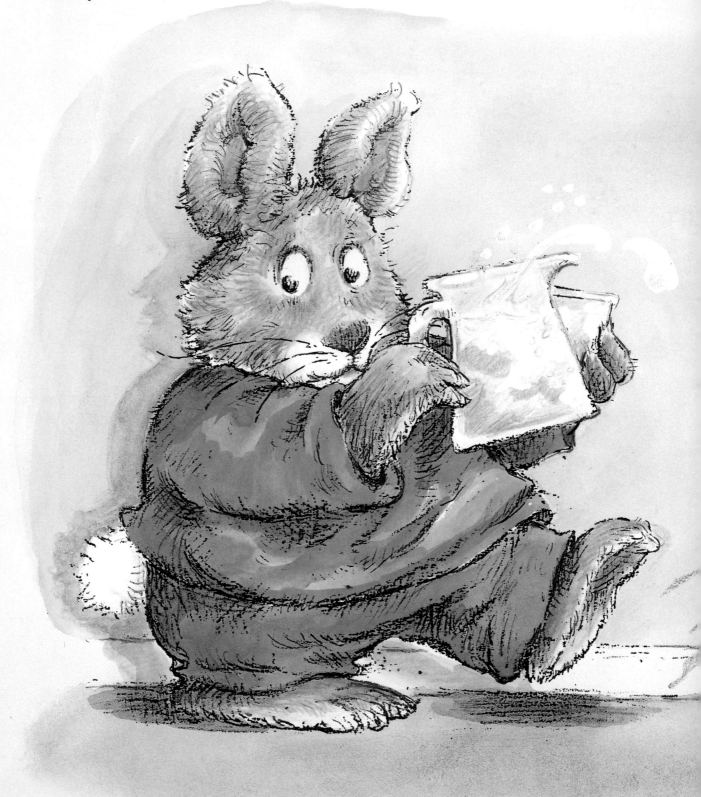

"Hic-hop," went Hyacinth Hop, as she hopped through the door.

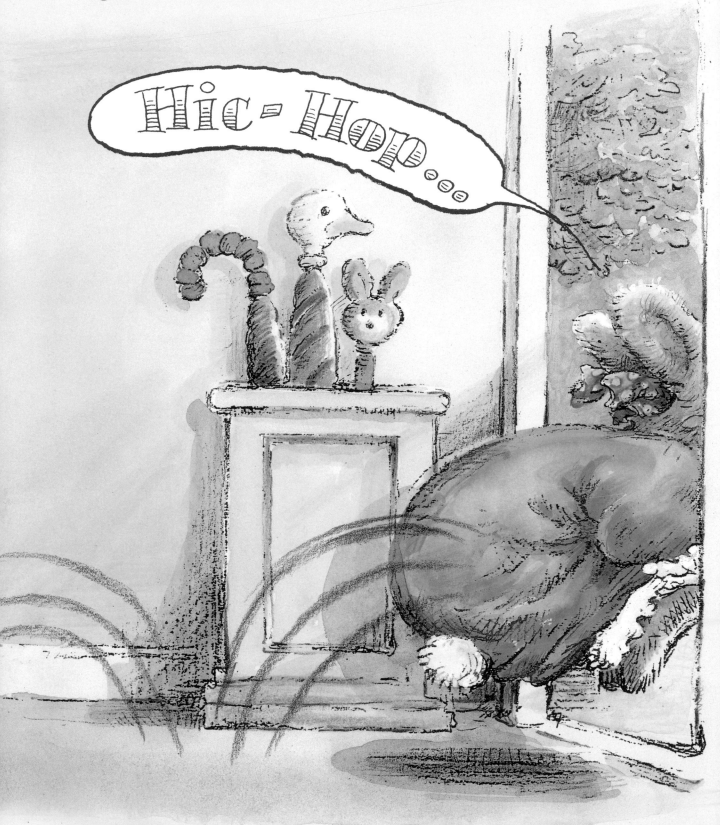

"Standing on the head is a cure - round you go Hyacinth."

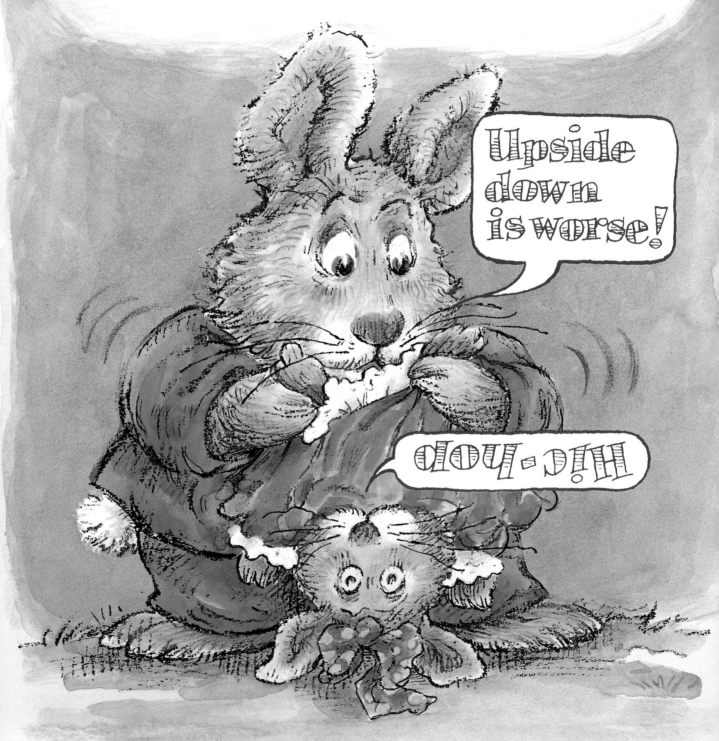

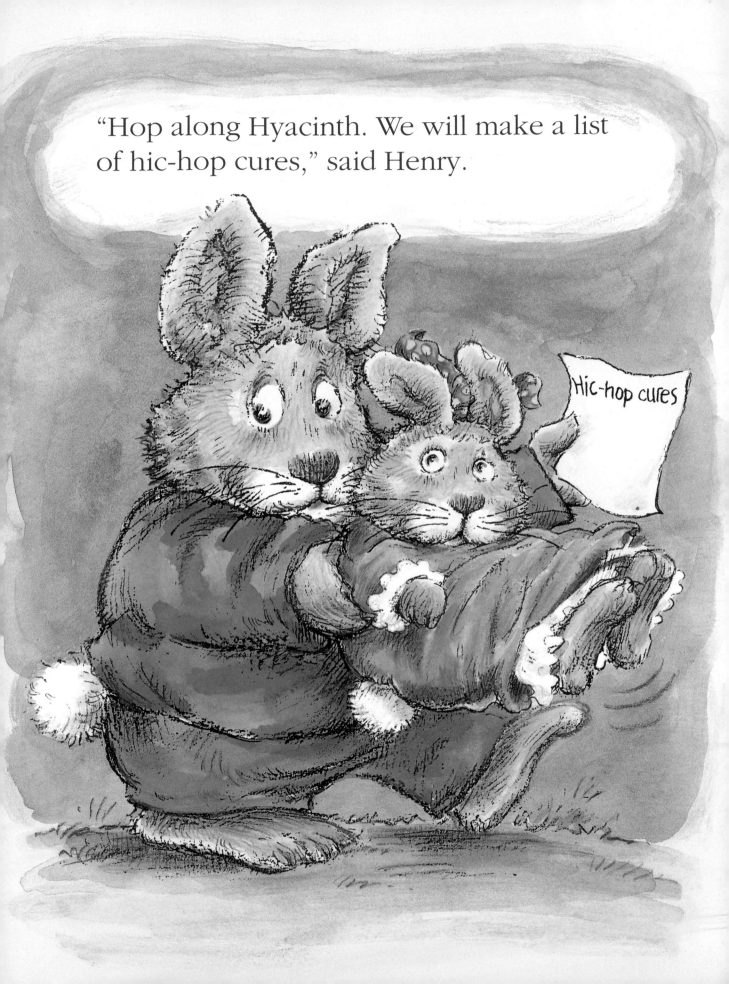

"Hop along Hyacinth. We will make a list of hic-hop cures," said Henry.

"A good dose of salts," said Dad. "That is a cure for the hic-hops."

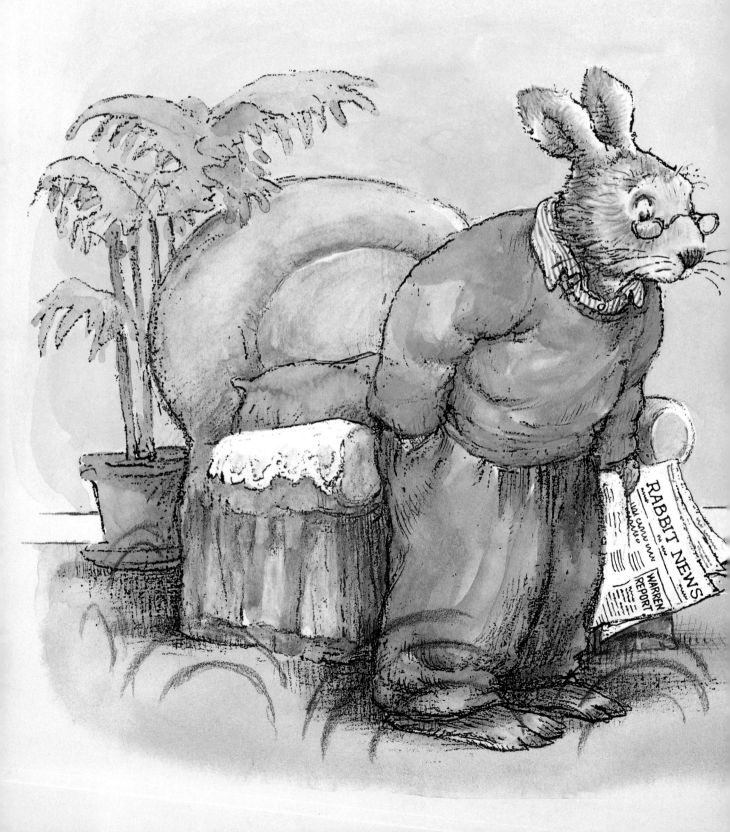

"Syrup of figs and nutmeg will stop them," said Mum.

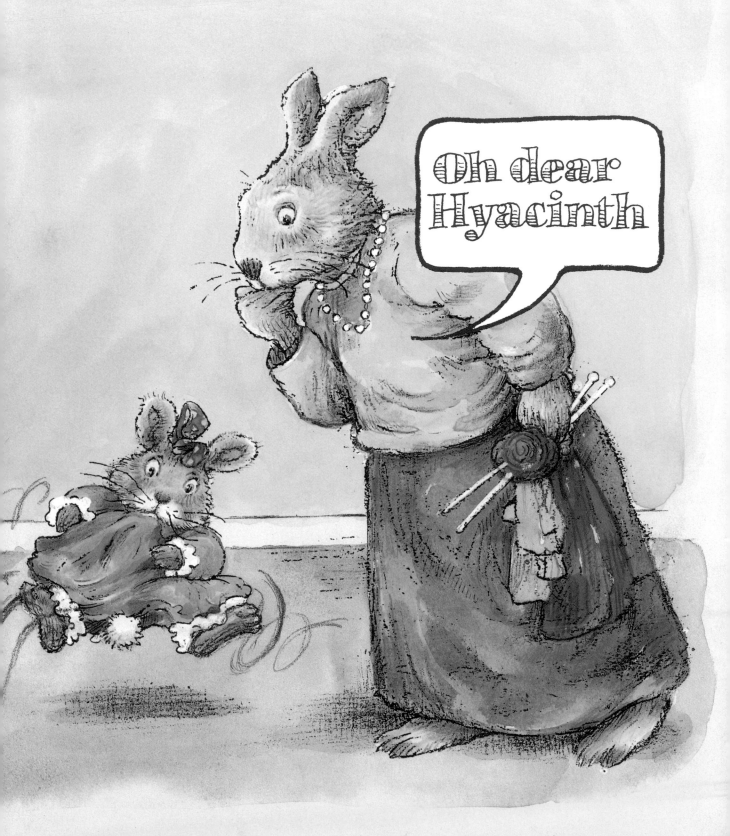

"We will go to market for a good dose of salts and syrup of figs with nutmeg."

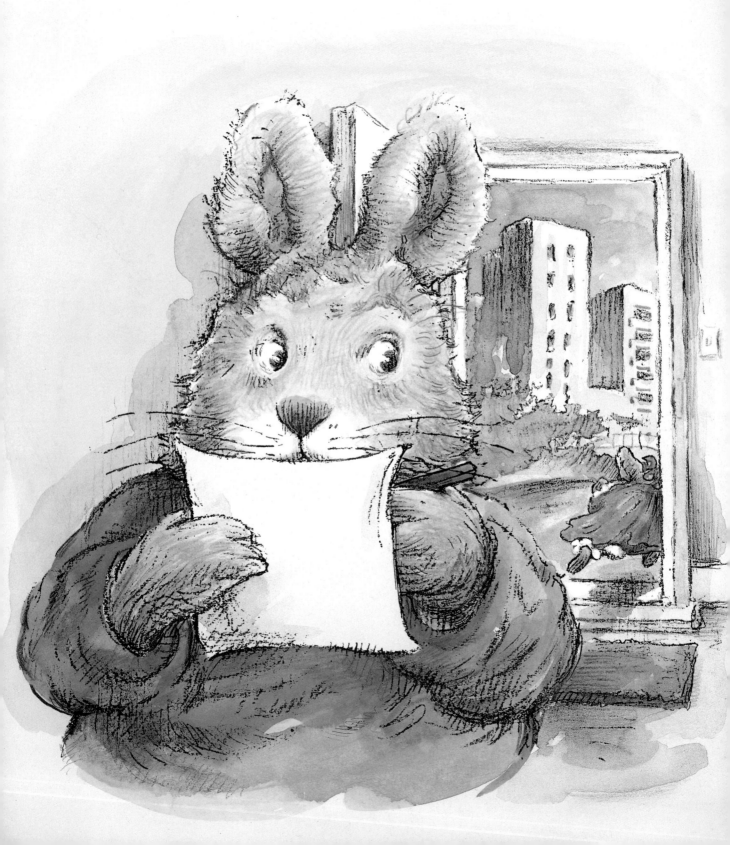

They met Uncle Bertram and Aunt Alice.
"A nice smelly gorgonzola will stop them," said
Uncle Bertram.

That girl has a problem

"Try ginger and vinegar first - that is a cure for hic-hops," said Aunt Alice.

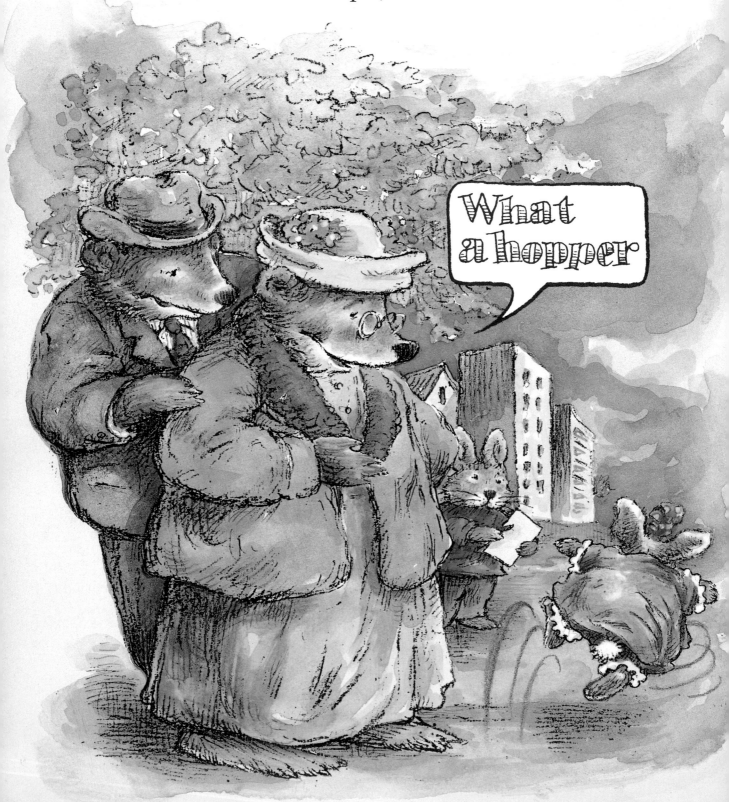

They hopped along to the shops.
Officer Riley was there. "Stewed rhubarb
and toothpaste, to be sure of a cure."

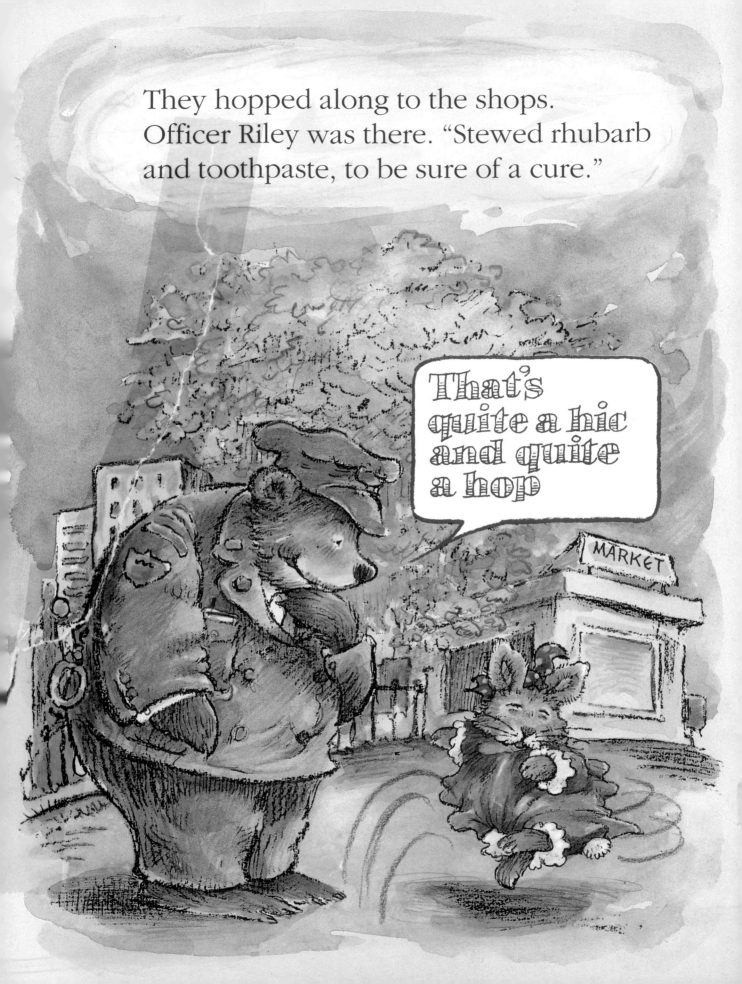

The list was full.

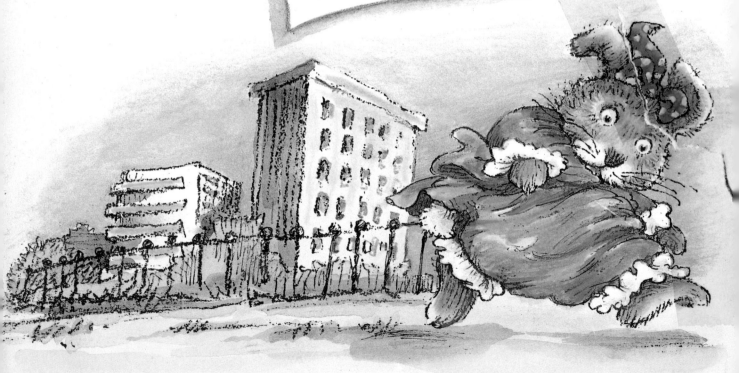

Hic-hop cures

1. A good dose of salts
2. Syrup of figs and nutmeg
3. A nice smelly gorgonzola
4. Ginger and vinegar
5. Stewed rhubarb and toothpaste

"Hic-hop," away to the shop went Hyacinth Hop.

"Hyacinth Hop has hic-hops. She will take these cures until the hic-hops stop," explained Henry.

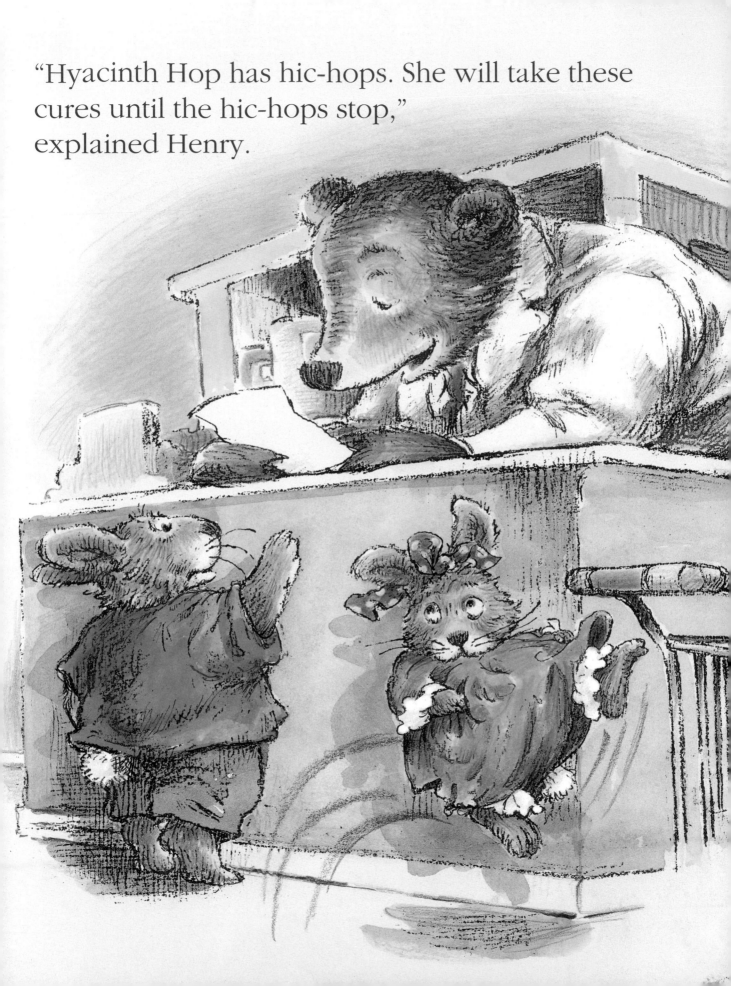

Hyacinth looked once, hopped twice...

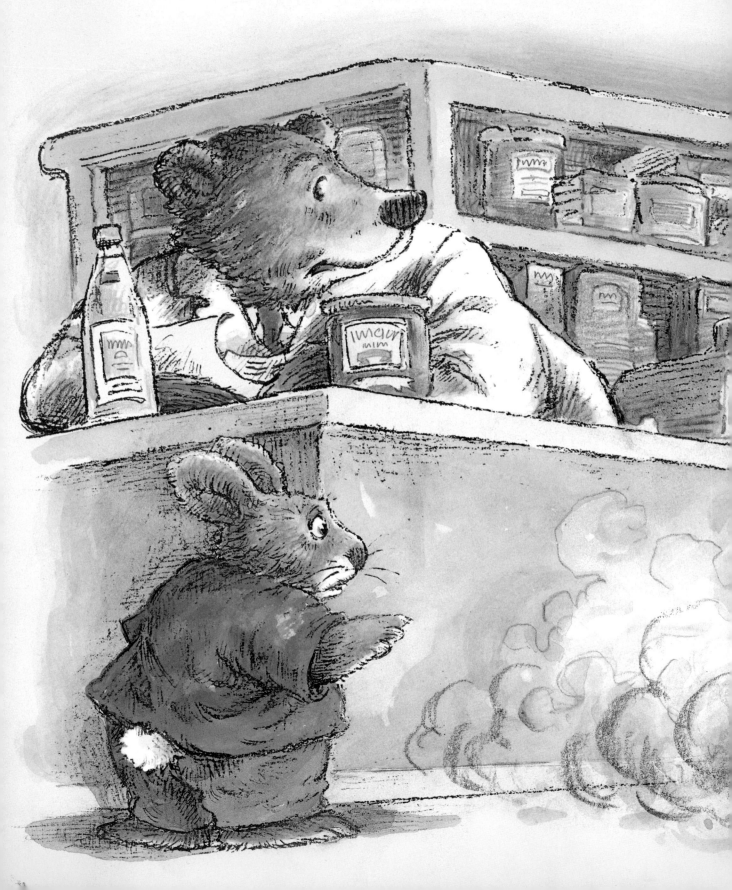

and was off!

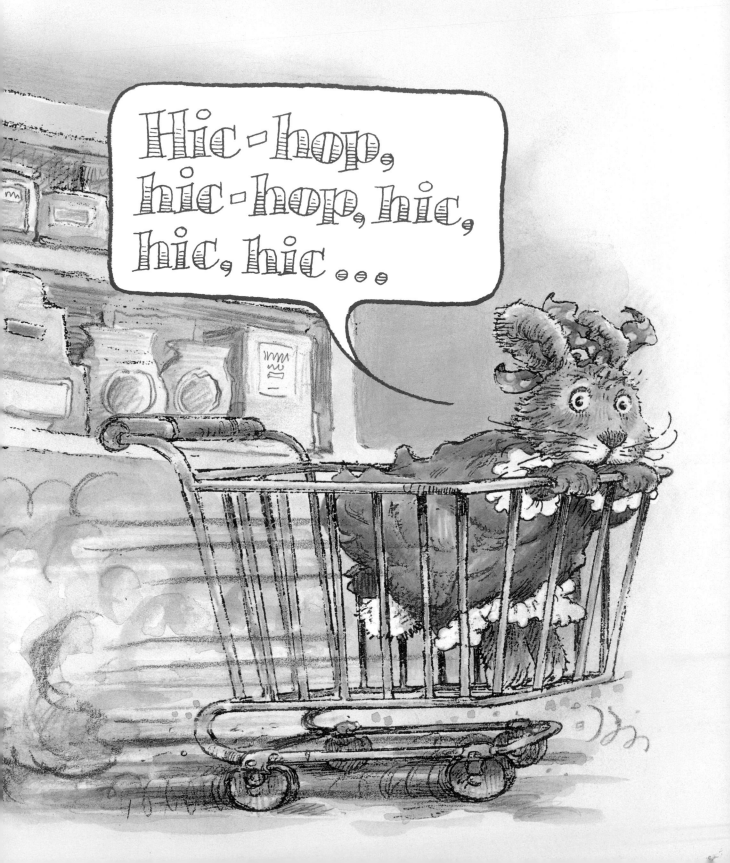

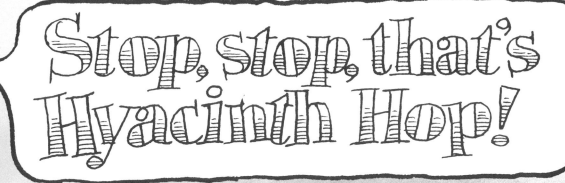

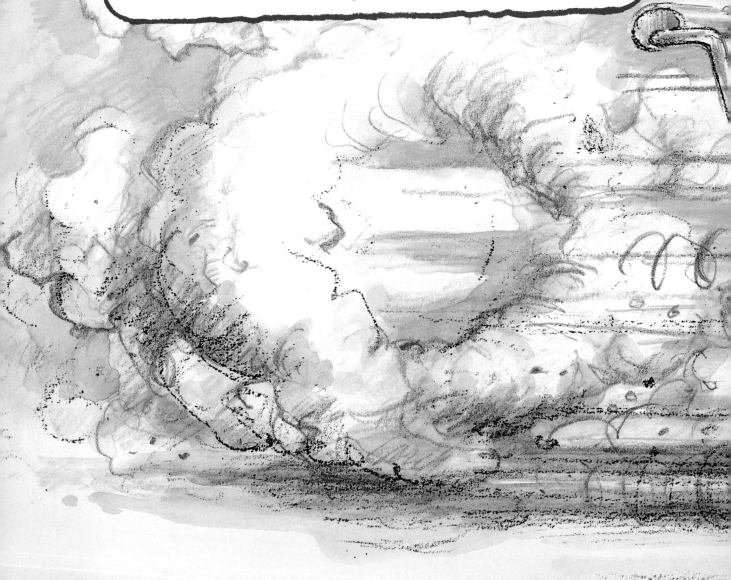

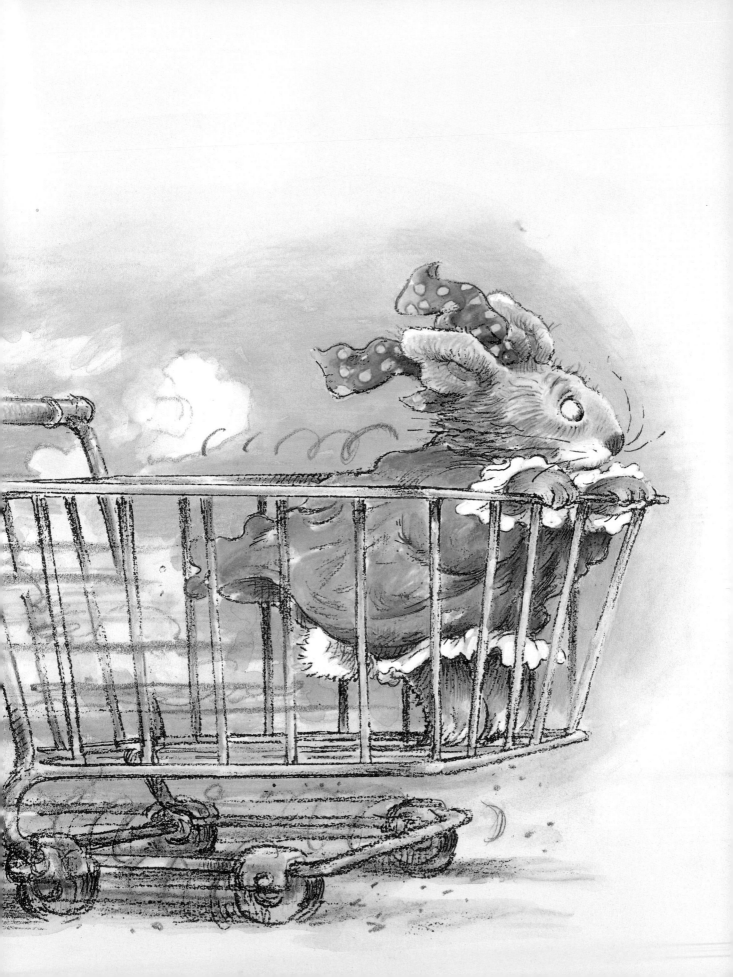

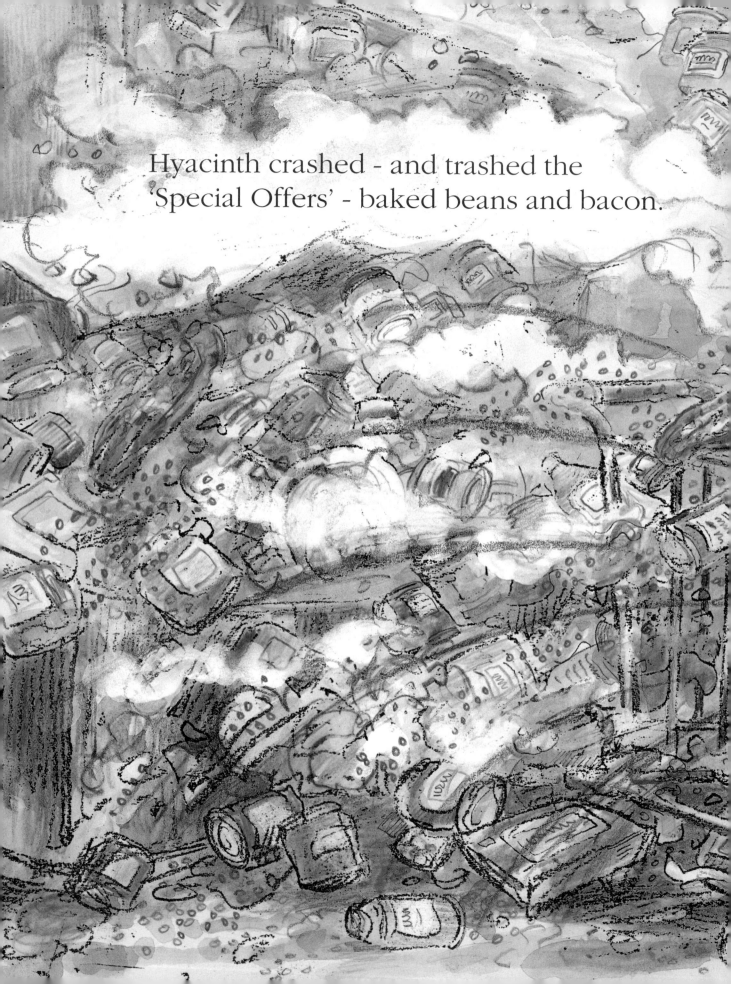

Hyacinth crashed - and trashed the
'Special Offers' - baked beans and bacon.

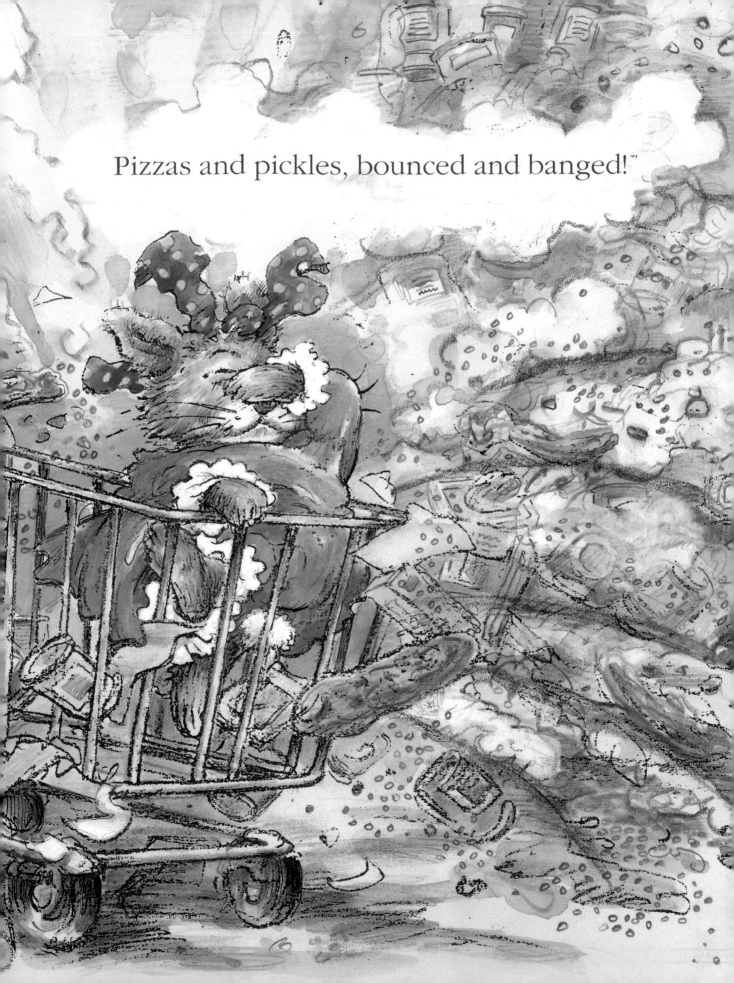

Pizzas and pickles, bounced and banged!

What a shock!
Hyacinth rolled to a stop, without a hic, without a hop.
Everyone looked at Hyacinth Hop - and waited...

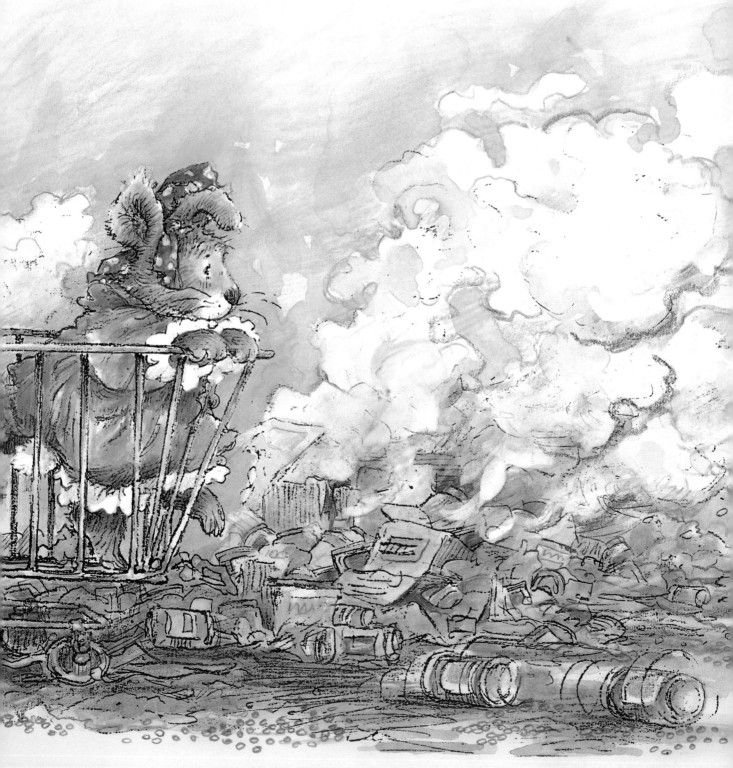

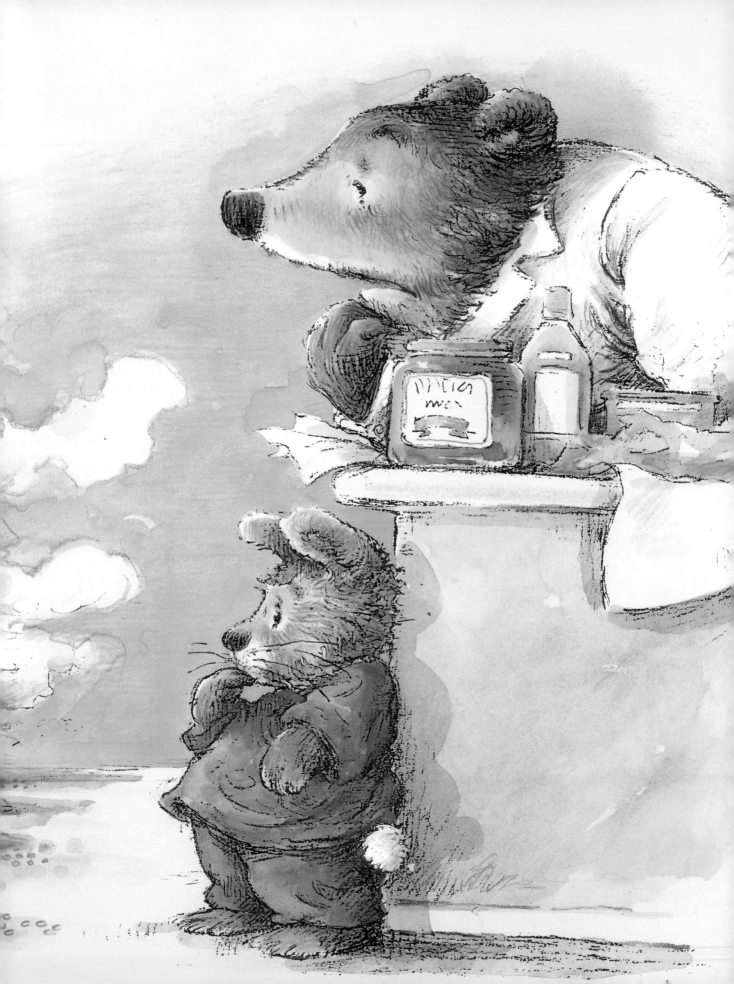

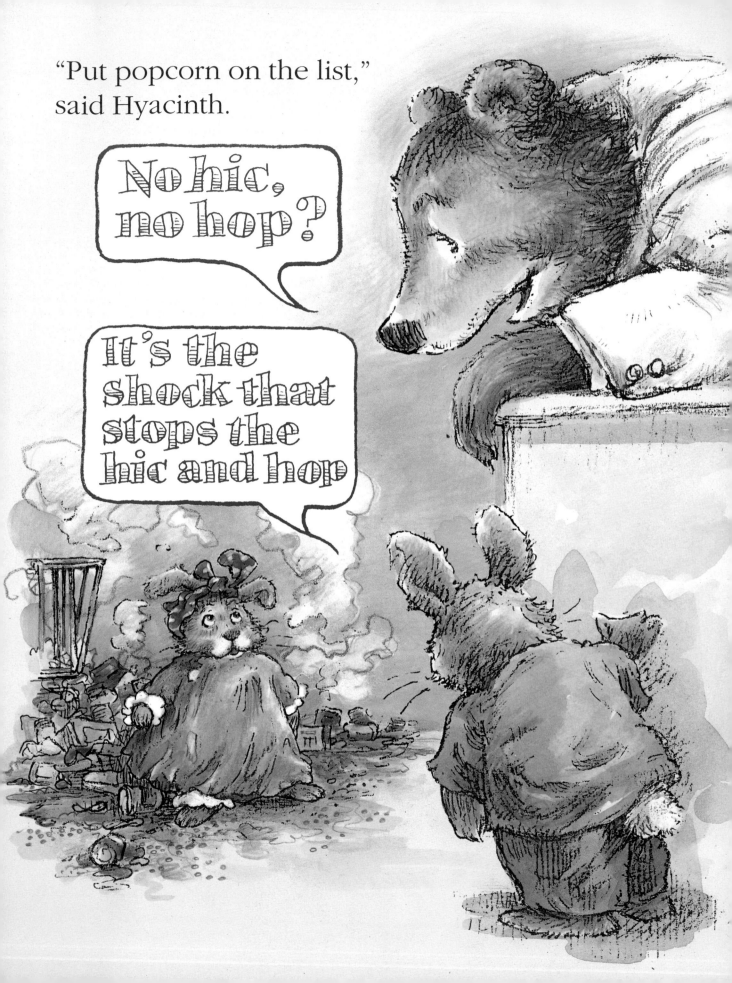

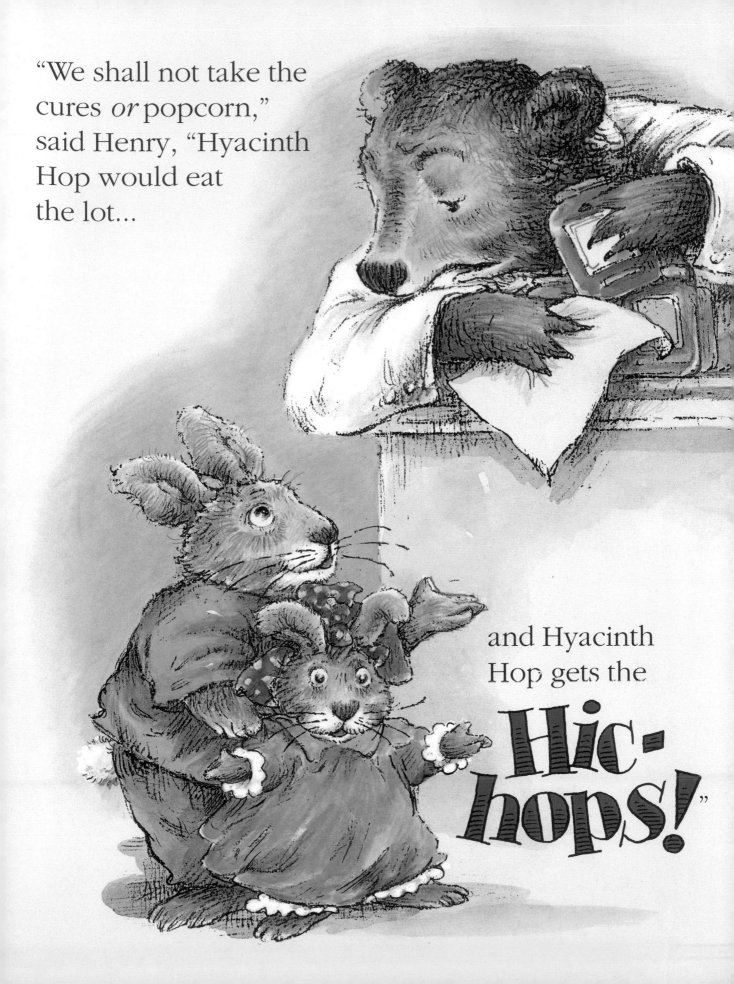

"We shall not take the cures *or* popcorn," said Henry, "Hyacinth Hop would eat the lot...

and Hyacinth Hop gets the

Hic-hops!"